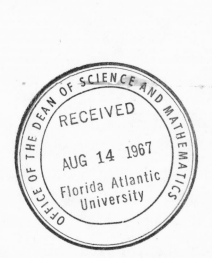

TEXTBOOK
OF
MEDICAL
PARASITOLOGY

TEXTBOOK
OF
MEDICAL
PARASITOLOGY

Haig H. Najarian, Ph.D.

Associate Professor of Biology,
University of Maine in Portland;
Formerly Consultant in Parasitic Diseases,
World Health Organization;
Assistant Professor of Microbiology,
The University of Texas Medical Branch;
Medical Zoologist, World Health Organization;
Assistant Professor of Biology, Boston University;
Associate Research Parasitologist, Parke, Davis & Co.;
Assistant Professor of Biology, Northeastern University;
Part-Time Instructor of Biology, Wayne State University.

The Williams & Wilkins Company

BALTIMORE · 1967

Illustrations by
MARTHA MILES GORDON

To the memory of my father,

HAGOP M. NAJARIAN,

who taught—and lived by—human dignity.

PREFACE

The purpose of this book is to provide a practical combination text and laboratory guide that can be easily read and used for a course in medical parasitology or medical zoology. Although there are several excellent parasitology textbooks, few would argue that these can be read and assimilated in the time usually allotted in medical curricula. Moreover, there are books intended to be used both as a laboratory guide and text, but these fall short in one respect or another. It is hoped that the manner of presentation of this book will circumvent many of the problems resulting from separate laboratory directions and text; that it will permit and induce the student to move comfortably through the pertinent aspects of medical parasitology; and finally, that it will provide him a basis for future utilization of his experience.

This book is written almost exclusively from the medical student's viewpoint, although it should be also useful to physicians, medical technologists, paramedical interests, and even for biology students to whom parasitology is taught from the medical standpoint. The usual medical student does not care about classification, because it has no practical use for him. He has no interest in zoological details that have no connection with a case. Moreover, although citations please the teacher of parasitology (especially if some allude to him), the medical student does not usually look up the elaborate references that are usually listed at the end of a chapter. The position is taken that the medical student simply wants to know the answers to certain basic questions:

1. What clinical picture might suggest a case of parasitism?
2. How did the patient become infected?
3. What happens in the body of an infected case?
4. How can diagnosis be established?
5. How should the case be treated?
6. What counsel can be given in terms of follow-up or prevention of future infection?

A biologist understandably may not agree with this limited point of view, but he ought at least to understand it both for its practical value and in the context of the small part medical parasitology has in the average medical school curriculum. Whatever the total postural web of the art and science of medicine may be, certainly a large part of it involves the practical approach to health. It is with all this in mind that this book is written, and if it lacks the usual definitive features one is used to, it is because of the chosen, limited approach. The hope is that it will help the student answer his realistic questions.

Since the initial patient-physician contact is brought about by signs and symptoms in a patient, the order of chapters in the book is not based on the phylogenetic approach. Rather, the arrangement of chapters is mostly in relation to the general areas of the body affected by parasitism. In those infections in which more than one area may be involved (and/or when the effects may be protean), the infection is considered in that category in which it is felt it would have the highest frequency in terms of symptomatology.

After some introductory remarks on the groups of parasites and a list of useful books in the field of medical parasitology, the chapter on *Integumentary Parasites and Venomous Animals* considers animal organisms associated with signs and symptoms of the integument and subcutaneous areas of patients. These include such animals as arthropods, protozoa, various types of worm infections, snakebite, and stings of jellyfish and rays. The chapter on *Intestinal Parasites* considers those parasites whose infections result mostly in gastrointestinal signs and symptoms, and the chapter on *Genitourinary Parasites* deals with the two most frequent genitourinary parasites. The chapter on *Tissue Parasites* includes those parasitic infections in which the signs and symptoms are primarily of various internal tissues and organs (excluding the gut). The parasitic infections contained in the chapter on *Vascular Parasites* have a profound effect on various parts of the vascular system and associated organs. Another common feature of this group of organisms is that the chief approach to diagnosis is by means of the stained blood smear.

For each of the infections, bites or stings (regardless of the chapter in which it is included) the sequence involves the clinical picture in the patient; the life cycle of the organism—particularly in the body; the means of diagnosis and treatment; post-treatment advice; and a few selected references. Most of the references are of a clinical nature, and therefore of the type that would have some attraction for further reading. It is felt that this order of presentation might approach simulation of the sequence of events that occur between a physician and patient in a given case.

For those students using this book as a laboratory guide, it is suggested that after reading the section on the clinical picture, the laboratory can be accomplished by the study of those materials relating and pertinent in the life cycle and diagnosis sections. This may be followed by reading the sections on treatment and post-treatment advice, in order to get a unified package from the exercise.

The last chapter (*Diagnosis and Treatment*) of the book includes summary comments on when parasites ought to be considered in a patient, how laboratory diagnosis is approached, and information on an alphabetical list of drugs mentioned in the respective sections of the text. Since it seems far more practical to learn what chemotherapeutic agents are useful rather than memorizing their dosages (which are soon forgotten), the dosage therapy as well as toxicity data are given in the final chapter rather than the respective sections of the book.

The illustrations were executed by Martha Miles Gordon, with whom it was a pleasure to work. Almost all were drawn from gross specimens or microscopic slides. The approach used in the drawings was to attempt to give a realistic *total* impression that could be observed by the student without great difficulty, rather than emphasizing structures that rarely are observable in an average preparation studied for a short time.

Appreciation is extended to Professor E. G. Nauck, and Georg Thieme Verlag, Stuttgart, for permission to reproduce their color plate of malaria parasites; to Leone Barnes, who typed the first two drafts of the manuscript; and to Dick M. Hoover and the staff of The Williams and Wilkins Company for complete cooperation in the completion of the book.

Acknowledgment is also directed to the almost one thousand sophomore medical students at the University of Texas Medical Branch (1960–66) for indicating (directly or indirectly) the kind of book they would consider useful.

Finally, the writer would welcome notification of errors and appreciate suggested changes that might make the book more suitable for its intention.

Portland, Maine   HAIG H. NAJARIAN

CONTENTS

chapter one

INTRODUCTION

Parasitology may be considered as a study of those animals possessing a certain way of life in which habitat is the chief factor. It is common knowledge that animals exist and satisfy their vital needs in just about every conceivable situation—on land, in the soil, in all types of aquatic environments, in the air, and in and on nonliving structures. It is therefore not surprising that many types of animals exist *on* and *within* other animals. Parasitism is an association between two animals in which the *parasite* becomes dependent upon, and usually produces some kind of injury to, its *host*. Just as democracy is a concept and therefore a matter of degree, parasitism is a conceptual degree of association of two animals.

There are over a million animal species, and the vast majority of them are of the invertebrate or nonbackboned type. Although there are some parasitic species in almost every taxonomic category of animals, those of medical importance belong to the following five groups: *protozoans*; *trematodes* (or *flukes*); *cestodes* (or *tapeworms*); *nematodes* (or *roundworms*); and *arthropods*. In addition to some arthropods, certain other animals introduce toxins from their bites and stings. A diversity of biological forms, such as jellyfish, snakes, spiders, scorpions and caterpillars, are included in this group. Although this arbitrary category of *venomous animals* is not parasitic in the usual sense of the word, it has considerable medical significance.

Protozoans

The vital needs of the usually microscopic protozoans take place within the confines of a single cell. Because these organisms mostly

1

have a single nucleus in their complete cytoplasm, they are often spoken of as unicellular organisms. But since the concept of a cell involves an anatomical and physiologic unit of a multicellular organism, the protozoa are probably better conceived of as acellular organisms in contrast to all other animals which are multicellular. One finds them referred to in both ways, but the chief point to realize is that they are organismic, and their being considered either as acellular or cellular is a question of human creation and depends on how interested one is in zoologic grammar and biologic concepts.

Just as multicellular organisms have tissues and organs for performing various vital functions, protozoa have specialized areas of their anatomy for specific functions—and these are referred to as *organelles.* The grouping of protozoans into class categories is based chiefly on the kind of locomotor organelles or the general lack of them.

Flagellates are characterized by the *flagellum* organelle of locomotion, which is composed of axial filaments plus a protoplasmic sheath continuous with the cytoplasm (Fig. 1A). Flagellates are the most primitive of animal types, and some share characteristics with certain types of plant organisms. Although there is a variety of forms, those of medical significance parasitize blood and tissue, the genitourinary tract, and the intestine of man.

Amebae utilize *pseudopodia* for locomotion. These structures are

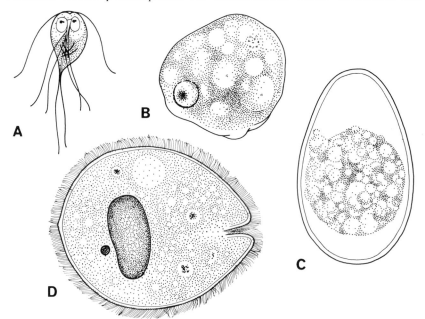

Fig. 1. Examples of four groups of protozoa: (A) *Giardia,* a flagellate; (B) *Entamoeba,* an ameba; (C) *Isospora,* a sporozoan; (D) *Balantidium,* a ciliate.

temporary protrusions of the cytoplasm (Fig. 1B). Although these protozoa exist in all kinds of ecologic situations and several exist in man, there is only one species which produces profound injury to the human gut and other tissues.

Sporozoans are usually extremely small, obligate parasites of cells of the vascular system, gut and other organs. Among other features, they are characterized by the general *absence* of locomotor organelles except during certain stages of their complicated life cycles (Fig. 1C). Those important to human medicine parasitize cells of the vascular system and other organs.

Ciliates move by means of organelles called *cilia,* which are structurally similar to flagella, except that they are very much shorter and extremely numerous on an organism (Fig. 1D). Only one species has medical significance, parasitizing the human gut, and even this species is not very prevalent in people.

Flatworms

These multicellular organisms include the *trematodes* (or *flukes*) and the *cestodes* (or *tapeworms*), all of which are parasitic. The worms vary in size from only a few mm to over several meters in length and are flat dorsoventrally. They usually have powerful muscular sucking discs for attachment and spines and hooks as armature. Much of their anatomy is composed of reproductive structures, most of them being hermaphroditic and having complicated life cycles.

Trematodes have a simple digestive tract, utilize snails as intermediate hosts for their larval forms, and parasitize the blood, lungs, liver and intestine of man. In hermaphroditic species (Fig. 2A) human infection occurs through ingestion of the cyst stage of the worm (on or in some other organism), whereas the bisexual blood flukes (Fig. 2B) infect man by skin penetration.

Tapeworms have several morphological features in common with trematodes but differ from the latter in that they are usually extremely long, completely lack a gut, do not utilize snails as intermediate hosts, have less complicated life cycles, and exist as a series of hermaphroditic, strobilate units (Fig. 2C). The head (or scolex) of most tapeworms bears sucker-like cups, hooks, and other armature for attachment (Figs. 2D & 2E). Adult tapeworms parasitize the human intestine, whereas the larval forms of some species seriously affect other parts of the human body.

Nematodes

These organisms are usually referred to as *roundworms* because of their cylindrical shape, and they vary in size from a few mm to over a

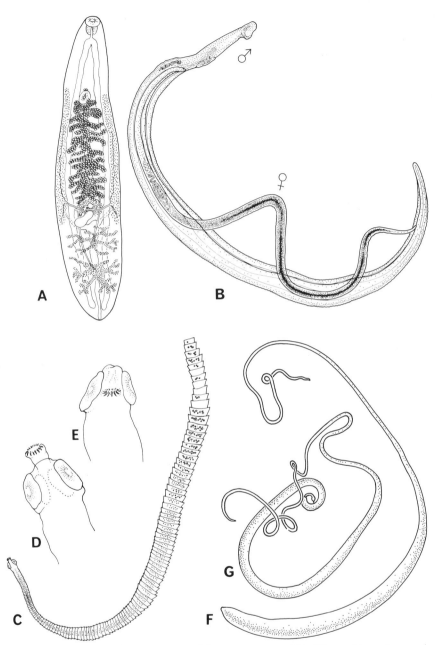

Fig. 2. Examples of some types of human worms: (A) *Clonorchis,* a hermaphroditic fluke; (B) *Schistosoma,* a pair of bisexual flukes; (C) *Hymenolepis,* a tapeworm; (D) and (E) *Hymenolepis,* two views of the head end, showing suckers, rostellum, and hooks; (F) and (G) *Trichuris,* a nematode (F, female; G, male).

meter in length. They have a tough cuticle and the sexes are separate, the female usually being considerably longer than the male (Figs. 2F & 2G). The vast majority are free-living in soil and water, but many parasitize plant and animal organisms. Those of medical importance

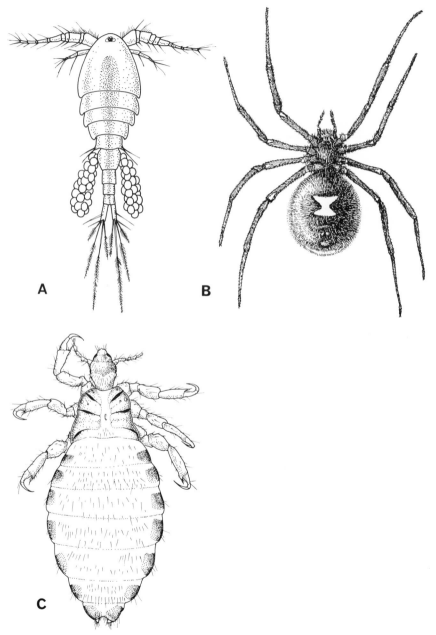

FIG. 3. Examples of some types of arthropods: (A) *Cyclops*, a crustacean; (B) *Latrodectus*, an arachnid; (C) *Pediculus*, an insect.

are found in the intestinal tract, vascular system, and other tissues, and—based on the number of cases—are the most important group of human parasites.

Arthropods

This is by far the largest group of animals—characterized by body segmentation, an exoskeleton, and paired, jointed appendages. While there are several subgroups in this collection of animals, very few classes of arthropods are of medical importance in terms of actual parasites or as transmitters of other disease organisms.

Crustaceans are a large, diverse, aquatic group of gill-breathing arthropods and include such familiar examples as crabs, crayfish, lobsters, barnacles and copepods (Fig. 3A). Some of them act as intermediate hosts for certain parasites.

Arachnids include the spiders, scorpions, ticks and mites, this group having adapted mostly to a terrestrial mode of life. These arthropods are characterized by having no antennae, 4 pairs of appendages in the adult stage, and the head and thorax usually fused into a single shield—the cephalothorax (Fig. 3B). They are air-breathers by several different mechanisms. While many are actual human parasites, others simply serve as vectors for a variety of microbial diseases.

Insects are mostly a terrestrial and aerial group of arthropods and include animals commonly referred to as "bugs," such as mosquitoes, fleas, roaches, wasps, beetles, moths, butterflies and lice. They have 1 pair of antennae, 3 pairs of appendages, and either 1, 2 or no pairs of wings. The insect body is divided into three parts: the head, thorax and abdomen (Fig. 3C). The medical importance of any insect is related to its way of life—particularly its mouthparts and its feeding habits. Certain insects transmit pathogens with no multiplication or cyclic development of the parasite, whereas in other insects the parasite undergoes either some metamorphosis and/or multiplies its numbers. Finally, many insects are important in terms of the hypersensitivity reactions of patients to their bites and stings.

GENERAL REFERENCES IN PARASITOLOGY

Ash, J. E., and Spitz, S. 1945. *Pathology of Tropical Diseases. An Atlas.* 350 pp., W. B. Saunders Company, Philadelphia.

Belding, D. L. 1965. *Textbook of Parasitology.* 3rd Ed., 1374 pp., Appleton-Century-Crofts, Inc., New York.

Brown, H. W., and Belding, D. R. 1964. *Basic Clinical Parasitology.* 2nd Ed., 318 pp., Appleton-Century-Crofts, Inc., New York.

Brooks, T. J., Jr. 1963. *Essentials of Medical Parasitology.* 359 pp., The Macmillan Company, New York.

Burrows, R. B. 1965. *Microscopic Diagnosis of the Parasites of Man.* 328 pp., Yale University Press, New Haven.

Cahill, K. M. 1964. *Tropical Diseases in Temperate Climates.* 225 pp., J. B. Lippincott Company, Philadelphia.

Chandler, A. C., and Read, C. P. 1961. *Introduction to Parasitology.* 10th Ed., 822 pp., John Wiley & Sons, New York.

Chatterjee, K. D. 1964. *Parasitology (Protozoology and Helminthology in Relation to Clinical Medicine).* 5th Ed., 208 pp., Calcutta - 26: 6, Amrita Banerjee Road, Kalighat, India.

Cheng, T. C. 1964. *The Biology of Animal Parasites.* 727 pp., W. B. Saunders Company, Philadelphia.

Faust, E. C., Beaver, P. C., and Jung, R. C. 1962. *Animal Agents and Vectors of Human Disease.* 2nd Ed., 485 pp., Lea & Febiger, Philadelphia.

Faust, E. C., and Russell, P. F. 1964. *Craig and Faust's Clinical Parasitology.* 7th Ed., 1099 pp., Lea & Febiger, Philadelphia.

Gordon, R. M., and Lavoirpierre, M. M. 1962. *Entomology for Students of Medicine.* 424 pp., F. A. Davis Company, Philadelphia.

Herms, W. B., and James, M. T. 1961. *Medical Entomology.* 5th Ed., 615 pp., The Macmillan Company, New York.

Hoare, C. A. 1949. *Handbook of Medical Protozoology.* 334 pp., Baillière, Tindall and Cox, London.

Horsfall, W. R. 1962. *Medical Entomology, Arthropods and Human Disease.* 465 pp., The Ronald Press Company, New York.

Hunter, G. W., Frye, W. W., and Swartzwelder, J. C. 1966. *A Manual of Tropical Medicine.* 4th Ed., 931 pp., W. B. Saunders Company,

Larsh, J. E., Jr. 1964. *Outline of Medical Parasitology.* 342 pp., McGraw-Hill Book Company, New York.

Markell, E. K., and Voge, M. 1965. *Medical Parasitology.* 2nd Ed., 317 pp., W. B. Saunders Company, Philadelphia.

Noble, E. R., and Noble, G. A. 1964. *Parasitology, the Biology of Animal Parasites.* 2nd Ed., 724 pp., Lea & Febiger, Philadelphia.

Sawitz, W. G. 1956. *Medical Parasitology.* 2nd Ed., 342 pp., McGraw-Hill Book Company, New York.

Spencer, F. M., and Monroe, L. S. 1961. *The Color Atlas of Intestinal Parasites.* 142 pp., Charles C. Thomas, Springfield, Illinois.

Swellengrebel, N. H., and Sterman, M. M. 1961. *Animal Parasites in Man.* 652 pp., D. Van Nostrand Company, Princeton, New Jersey.

Watson, J. M. 1960. *Medical Helminthology.* 487 pp., Baillière, Tindall and Cox, London.

chapter two

INTEGUMENTARY PARASITES AND VENOMOUS ANIMALS

The human integument, in addition to its operational functions, is the first line of defense toward the outside environment. One may think of the integument as a territorial line. Excepting those parasites which enter the body through one of the orifices, the parasite entering the skin is met with various defense factors. The outcome of this meeting is an algebraic sum of the body defense and the invasive machinery of the parasite. The nature of some parasites is such that they enter the body via the integument with little or no difficulty, take up various locations in the body, develop to maturity, and reproduce. Their progeny then pass out of the body by various life cycle routes, via insect transmission, or in some cases end up as so-called blind alley infections. Although this is the usual pattern, there is a whole spectrum of possible events when contact is made with the integument.

The array of possibilities is exhibited mostly by the arthropod group of animals. Contact may be short in time and involve nothing more than mechanical injury to tissue. More often there is toxic injury due to materials released during an insect bite. Some arthropods actually invade tissue and spend some or most of their lives in that location. In contacts with other species there develop both local and general hypersensitive reactions on multiple exposures to bites or stings. Allergy may also develop to contact or to inhalation of some body substance.

Of severe consequence in some is the release of toxins, which may act in a local or systemic fashion. Toxins are involved not only in

9

some arthropods, but in several other invertebrate and vertebrate animals, notably jellyfish and snakes.

Some worm parasites never get much beyond the skin, while other species penetrate and mature in deeper tissue.

Of probably outstanding importance is the fact that many arthropods in their temporary contacts of feeding off the human body act as vectors in the transmission of a variety of disease-producing agents —namely, viruses, rickettsiae, protozoa, and helminths.

Many of the organisms considered in this chapter are not parasites in the sense that protozoa and worms of man are, but rather their outstanding effects on the body are either in a transient fashion or due to such features as hypersensitivity and toxins (from bites and stings) and also to the fact of their acting as mechanical or biologic vectors in the transmission of pathogenic agents.

The theme that groups these organisms together is that the initial clinical effects are with the human integument. Visual recognition of the organism is of prime importance in suspecting what is wrong with the patient and also in predicting the course of events which may follow, as well as the necessary action one ought to take. In cases where there has been only temporary contact of the patient with the animal, one must rely on indirect evidence (such as the clinical picture, bite or sting marks) in making an intelligent diagnosis.

TICKS

Hard Ticks

Soft Ticks

Clinical Picture. Tickbite may result in any of three types of situations: mechanical injury to the integument; a type of paralysis due to substances released by the tick during feeding; and transmission of various rickettsial, viral, bacterial and spirochetal diseases of humans and other animals.

Ticks attach at any point on the body, and there is an inflammatory reaction around the anterior head-like structure. There may be itching around the erythema of the lesion, although the initial bite is not painful, and a patient rarely knows that he has a tick until a few hours after the contact. Some ticks stay attached for only a few hours, while others may suck blood for several days and then drop off. The wound may become secondarily infected and necrotic.

In some patients (especially young children) when the tick bites in apposition to the central nervous system, there develops a condition called *tick paralysis*. This is characterized by an ascending motor

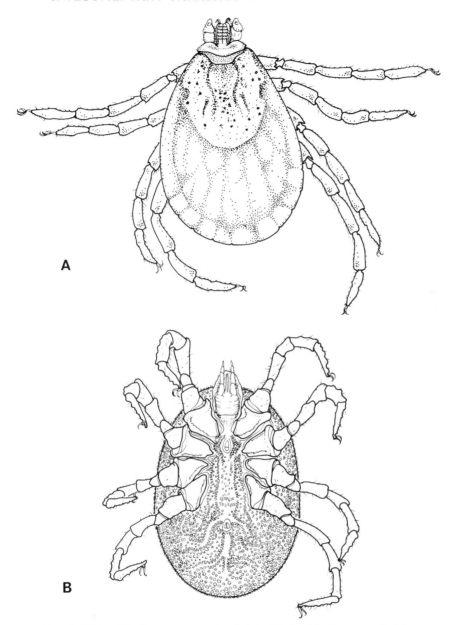

FIG. 4. Ticks: (A) *Dermacentor*, a hard tick; (B) *Ornithodorus*, a soft tick.

paralysis, fever, and general intoxication, leading to various respiratory difficulties. The condition may be fatal. The paralysis is due to toxic substances released in the saliva of the tick, rather than an infectious agent.

Ticks are also involved in the transmission of bacterial tularemia, the rickettsial spotted fevers, viral Colorado tick fever, spirochetal relapsing fever, and other pathogens. Since these diseases are discussed in other texts, they will not be considered here.

Life Cycle. A person is bitten by a tick because he happens to be at the right place at the right time. Ticks are not host specific and suck blood from a variety of large and small animals. The life cycle of these arthropods includes the egg, larva, nymph and adult stages. Although the latter three stages are all blood-suckers, the adult tick is the one that usually bites man. The number of blood meals, changes of host, and other aspects of the life cycle vary considerably, according to the tick species involved.

Diagnosis. Adult ticks (except when engorged) are flattened dorsoventrally, have 4 pairs of legs, and no visible segmentation of the body. There are two general types of ticks—the *soft ticks* and the *hard ticks.* Hard ticks (Fig. 4A) have a dorsal shield, and the mouthparts are visible when viewed from the dorsal aspect, whereas soft ticks lack the dorsal shield, and the mouthparts attach ventrally and are therefore not visible from the dorsal aspect (Fig. 4B). Ticks are cosmopolitan in geographic distribution. Since the clinician's interest is usually to know only if something is a tick, an entomologist or parasitologist should be consulted if further identification is desired.

Treatment. Early removal of the tick is of prime importance. This is accomplished by steady traction on the tick body by means of forceps or fingers. Some advise a drop of chloroform or ether on the tick before removal. The point is to remove all of the arthropod. If the anchored head breaks off, it should be removed surgically. The wound is treated with iodine or some other antiseptic agent.

Post-Treatment Advice. Patients requiring to work or travel in tick-infested areas should be advised to treat their clothes with repellants or use tick-proof clothing. Benzene hexachloride (Lindane) has proved to be a highly effective agent against both soft and hard ticks. It can be purchased as a spray, dust or dip.

SELECTED REFERENCES

Arthur, D. R. 1962. *Ticks and Disease,* 445 pp., Pergamon Press, London.
Hoogstraal, H. 1966. Ticks in relation to human diseases caused by viruses. *Ann. Rev. of Entomol., 11:* 261.
Rose, I. 1954. A review of tick paralysis. *J. Canad. Med. Assoc., 70:* 175.

MITES

Scabies mite	*Sarcoptes scabei*
Follicular mite	*Demodex folliculorum*
Chigger mite	trombiculid mite

Clinical Picture. The most characteristic feature resulting from mite contact with the human integument is varying degrees of dermatitis. Except in certain areas of the world, the role of mites in the transmission of disease pathogens is very minor compared to that of ticks. There is a considerable number of mite species which are normally associated with other vertebrates (such as birds, rodents and insects) and which may cause human dermatitis and itching upon biting a patient. However, all of these are of inconsequential medical importance, and the number of mites as true human parasites or presenting real medical problems is quite small.

Human mange (scabies or the seven-year itch) causes considerable tissue injury and reaction of the human integument. The human scabies mite lives in serpiginous tunnels made in the skin, resulting in erythema and intense itching. As the infection gets older, a generalized pruritic rash develops on the body. Uncontrollable scratching predisposes to secondary infections with pustules, scab development and eczemic scales.

The human follicular mite also has an obligate association with the human integument and parasitizes hair follicles and sebaceous glands. However, it causes relatively little difficulty, no dermatitis, but rather only localized keratitis or possibly blackhead formation.

Of considerable importance is the chigger mite (red bug or trombiculid mite). It is the larval stage of this arthropod that causes difficulty when coming into contact with human skin. It does not burrow but rather attaches by its mouthparts and feeds on tissue fluids. Its salivary fluid releases substances into human skin which result in very severe itching and dermatitis. Erythema develops around the bite, and secondary infection is not uncommon as a result of uncontrollable scratching.

Life Cycle. Patients become infected with scabies and the follicle mite by close personal contact with other infected individuals, whereas the normal habitat of chiggers is in brushy areas where these mites live on the ground. Mites are cosmopolitan in geographic distribution. The life cycle of most mites is similar to that of ticks, having an egg, larva, nymph and adult stage. The adult female scabies mite lays her eggs in skin burrows, and the larval and nymph stages which develop also burrow in the skin. The entire life cycle of the follicular mite takes place within hair follicles. In the chigger mite man simply serves as a temporary host for the larva before it drops or crawls off the skin and eventually develops into an adult mite.

Diagnosis. Recovery of the mite from the skin and its microscopic identification results in firm diagnosis. Most morphologic characteristics that apply to ticks also apply to mites, except that the latter are usually microscopic and hairy-looking. The nature of the lesions and their location on the body, as well as rash distribution, are also helpful in establishing the diagnosis. The female scabies mite and its eggs may be recovered from the end of the skin tunnels by a needle or skin

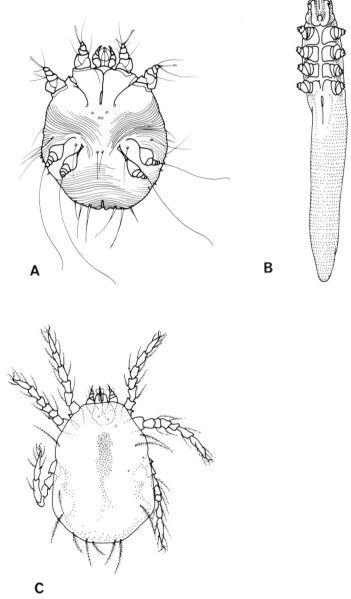

FIG. 5. Mites: (A) *Sarcoptes*, the scabies mite; (B) *Demodex*, the follicular mite; (C) trombiculid chigger mite larva.

scrapings. However, since the number of mites on a patient is usually small, they cannot always be successfully demonstrated. In such cases an itching rash in which the soles of the feet, palms of the hands, and face are not involved should always suggest scabies.

The scabies mite (Fig. 5A) is an oval, flattened, hairy arthropod, whereas the follicle mite (Fig. 5B) is an elongate, cylindrical, worm-like mite with 4 pairs of stubby legs and a nonhairy body. Since it is a larval mite, the chigger (Fig. 5C) has only 3 pairs of legs, and its body is covered with minute hairs.

Treatment. A soapy, scrubby bath is the first thing that is required. A single application of benzene hydrochloride (Lindane) ointment or a few applications of benzyl benzoate lotion is effective against scabies. The follicle mite is also cleared with Lindane ointment. Topical sulfur ointment is effective against chiggers. Palliatives may be required, as well as mercurial ointment for secondary infections.

Post-Treatment Advice. Patients who run occupational and avocational risks toward mite infections should be advised as to the use of such chemical repellants as chlordane.

SELECTED REFERENCES

Breckenridge, R. L. 1953. Infestation of the skin with *Demodex folliculorum. Amer. J. Clin. Pathol., 23:* 348.

Johnson, C. G., and Mellanby, K. 1942. The parasitology of human scabies. *Parasitology, 34:* 285.

Robinson, T. W. E. 1965. *Demodex folliculorum* and rosacea. *Arch. Dermatol., 92:* 542.

Russell, B. 1964. Parasitic infestations of the skin. *The Practitioner, 195:* 621.

LICE

Head and body louse	*Pediculus humanis*
Pubic louse	*Phthirus pubis*

Clinical Picture. Human lice are blood-suckers, and the general clinical picture depends on what part of the integument is involved and the sensitivity of the patient to the louse's saliva. The bite produces an elevated papule which results in intense itching. Dermatitis and urticaria may develop, and scratching may lead to secondary infection. Long involvement of the scalp may result in scaling and hair loss. In chronic cases of body lice the skin becomes thickened and hyperpigmented. Bluish spots may develop around the louse bites in the pubic region. The body louse transmits epidemic typhus, trench fever, and epidemic relapsing fever.

Life Cycle. Since human lice are highly host specific, patients become infested by close association with their fellow humans and/or their fomites. The geographic distribution of lice is cosmopolitan. The head louse lives attached usually to hairs at the back of the head, and the crab louse to the hairs, especially of the pubic region. Both of these lice lay their eggs (or nits) cemented to hairs in their respective locations. The favorite sites of the body louse are clothing fibers and hairs of the axilla and chest. The body louse cements her eggs to the fibers of clothing, especially in the seam region. Nymphs develop from the egg case and, after emerging, also suck blood until they are mature.

Diagnosis. Demonstration of lice and/or eggs from an itchy, scratchy patient establishes the diagnosis. The eggs or nits (Fig. 6C) are white, glistening, round objects and, in the case of head and pubic lice, are recovered from human hair, whereas those from the body louse are found from the patient's clothing. Human lice are wingless insects with a dorsoventrally flattened body. The 3 pairs of legs are well developed and have claws at their terminal ends. Whereas the bodies of head and body lice (Fig. 6B) are elongate, those of crab lice (Fig. 6A) are nearly as wide as they are long. The latter also have much better developed claws on their legs.

Treatment. Palliatives are given for the itching, and after a hot, soapy bath, Lindane ointment or lotion and DDT talcum is applied for getting rid of the lice. Shaving the hair of affected areas is also desirable. Boiling of the clothes is also necessary for a patient having body lice.

Post-Treatment Advice. Personal hygiene in the form of frequent bathing should be stressed, as well as repellants for persons who run a high risk of exposure in crowded conditions and situations.

SELECTED REFERENCES

Buxton, P. A. 1947. *The Louse, an Account of the Lice Which Infect Man, Their Medical Importance and Control.* 2nd Ed., Arnold, London.

Peck, S. M., Wright, W. H., and Gant, J. P. 1943. Cutaneous reactions due to the body louse. *J.A.M.A., 123:* 821.

Zinsser, H. 1935. *Rats, Lice, and History.* 301 pp., Little, Brown & Company, Boston.

BUGS

Bedbug   *Cimex lectularius*

Triatomid bugs $\begin{cases} \textit{Triatoma infestans} \\ \textit{Panstrongylus megistus} \\ \textit{Rhodnius prolixus} \end{cases}$

Clinical Picture. Bugs refer to insects of a particular sort, and included in this group are two which suck human blood—the bedbug and the triatomid bug. The outcome of a patient's being bitten depends on his sensitivity and the species of bug that bites. Neither bedbugs nor triatomid bugs are host specific.

Bedbugs inflict a bite which becomes erythemic and very itchy.

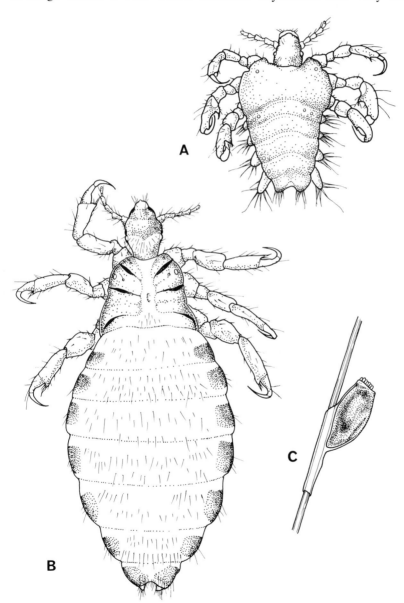

Fig. 6. Lice: (A) *Phthirus*, the pubic louse; (B) *Pediculus*, the head or body louse; (C) louse egg, or nit, attached to hair.

Some patients react more violently than others to the bug's saliva, and this results in hemorrhagic spots around the bite, dermatitis, and even urticaria. The bites and spots usually occur in a linear fashion.

The bites of some triatomid bugs are painless, while in others the saliva contains toxic materials which lead to pain, itching and swelling around the bite area. Triatomid bugs transmit Chagas' disease—to be described later.

Life Cycle. Both bedbugs and triatomid bugs are nocturnal in their feeding habits and will suck blood from most any mammal. A patient is bitten at night, usually when sleeping. The bedbug customarily feeds while on bedclothes or sheets, while the triatomid bug prefers to be on the integument while sucking blood. Liquid feces are released immediately after feeding and—in the case of triatomids—usually contaminate the lesion, making it an important vector of some pathogens. Although the bedbug experimentally can transmit a variety of pathogenic organisms, its feeding position is apparently a factor in its not playing a role in the transmission of human diseases. The eggs of each bug are laid in various crevices around the house. The nymphs which hatch are also blood suckers. Although the geographic distribution of bedbugs is cosmopolitan, that of triatomid bugs is confined to the Americas.

Diagnosis. Restlessness at night due to bites is suggestive of these

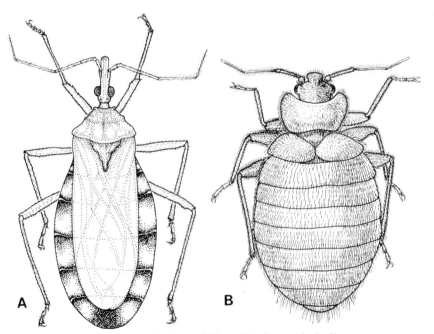

A   B

FIG. 7. Bugs: (A) a triatomid bug; (B) *Cimex*, the bedbug.

two bugs. Bedbugs (Fig. 7B) tend to bite in a linear fashion on the trunk and arms, whereas triatomid bugs bite with higher frequency on the face, especially around the mouth and eyes. Both bugs have a long proboscis which is folded ventrally under the body when not in use, and this one feature distinguishes them from other human insects. Triatomid bugs (Fig. 7A) also have the added characteristics of an elongate, pointed head and yellow or orange color markings on the body of many species. Bedbugs cannot fly, but the triatomids are aerial.

Treatment. Topical palliatives are given for the itching and antihistamines for possible dermatitis.

Post-Treatment Advice. Lindane spraying or DDT dusting should be advised for the home of the patient.

SELECTED REFERENCES

Johnson, C. G. 1941. The ecology of the bedbug, *Cimex lectularius* L., in Britain. *J. Hyg., 41:* 345.

Lavoirpierre, M. M., Dickerson, G., and Gordon, R. M. 1959. The manner in which triatomid bugs obtain a blood meal. *Ann. Trop. Med. & Parasitol., 53:* 235.

FLEAS

Human flea	*Pulex irritans*
Sand flea	*Tunga penetrans*

Clinical Picture. With one exception, fleas do not invade the human integument but rather suck blood in a similar fashion as other blood-sucking insects. The lesion from a flea bite is annoying, and the irritation caused by the flea's saliva may result in raised erythemic spots of various dermatologic conditions—depending on the sensitivity of the patient. Fleas have relatively low host specificity, and their real medical importance is in the transmission of various diseases, such as plague and endemic typhus.

The sand, or chigoe, flea is not known to transmit human pathogens, but it is the female of this flea which causes considerable damage to the human integument. Instead of laying eggs on the body or on the ground (as do other fleas), she burrows into the skin, sucks blood and lays her eggs. She becomes fatter, resulting in the protrusion of her rear end to the outside environment. The initial lesion develops a central black spot surrounded by a pale area. Secondary infection is common to the inflamed, painful, itchy lesion, and the whole affair can become quite serious.

Life Cycle. Since fleas will feed on practically any mammal, a pa-

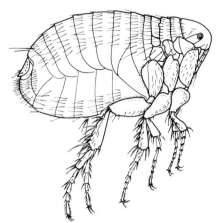

Fig. 8. *Pulex*, a human flea.

tient becomes bitten by circumstances of time and place, although certain factors are predisposing. There are certain species which occur mostly on man, although a patient may play host to those normally found associated with dogs, cats, rodents, hogs and other animals. Fleas lay white, glistening eggs which pass through a worm-like larval stage, followed by further development in a cocoon structure before reaching adult maturity. The eggs are laid in various locations—on the ground, in crevices of the house, in the nests of animals, and on pets. Because of their powerful legs, they can jump easily from one animal to another.

Diagnosis. A patient with annoying bites of unknown origin usually has a pet dog or cat. Most fleas have cosmopolitan geographic distribution. Eggs and larval stages can easily be recovered from the area where the family pet sleeps. Adult fleas are very distinctive-looking, wingless insects, and diagnosis of the arthropod is a relatively simple matter. The body of the flea (Fig. 8) is laterally compressed, there are 3 pairs of powerfully developed legs, and most species have pronounced eyes and backward-pointing spine-like structures on the body.

The relatively small, foreshortened sand flea is identified after excision from the lesion. An entomologist or parasitologist should be consulted for species determination.

Treatment. Palliatives are given for the itching and antihistamines for dermatitis. The sand flea must be removed surgically and the wound treated as a bacterial sore.

Post-Treatment Advice. Personal hygiene should be stressed in the case of human fleas, whereas in the case of nonhuman fleas, the question becomes one of control of fleas of pets, those of other animals, and rodent control. DDT or Lindane dusting is effective, and various repellants can be used when a patient runs a high risk of flea contact.

SELECTED REFERENCE

Reiss, F. 1966. Tungiasis in New York City. *Arch. Dermatol., 93:* 404.

FLIES

Mosquitoes	**Deer flies**
Sandflies	**Horse flies**
Black flies	**Stable flies**

There is a variety of flies (or *dipterans*) which constitute the outstanding group of medically-important arthropods. Their most important feature is their role in either the mechanical or biologic transmission of a variety of protozoal, bacterial, helminthic and viral diseases. These include African trypanosomiasis, malaria, filariasis and onchocerciasis, batonellosis, tularemia, and the viral encephalitides. The blood-sucking flies include the mosquitoes, sandflies, back flies, deer flies, and others, all of which transmit diseases to humans. Such dipterans as stable flies and horse flies also bite humans but are not known to transmit human pathogens. Of outstanding importance is the house fly, which certainly does not bite but nevertheless transmits a variety of viral, bacterial and protozoal infections to man. The following section deals with the blood-sucking group of flies only in terms of injury due to the bite and the effects of salivary substances introduced into the human integument.

Clinical Picture. The effect of fly bites depends on the type of fly and the sensitivity of the patient. Some bites (sandflies) are immediately painful, whereas others (deer flies) become painful only after several hours. The bites of most flies are of minor consequence. On the average there is some degree of erythema, itching and swelling. Secondary infection may follow as a result of scratching. Sensitive patients may exhibit allergic reactions such as urticaria, accompanied by severe itching, fever and nausea.

Life Cycle. A patient is bitten by circumstance. The blood-sucking flies usually have a certain period of the day or night when they actively feed, and they breed in various ecologic situations. Most flies have a wide geographic distribution in nature, and although their life cycle stages are often pertinent to their classification, they are not of interest or value to the average clinician.

Diagnosis. Medical attention is usually not sought unless the bite

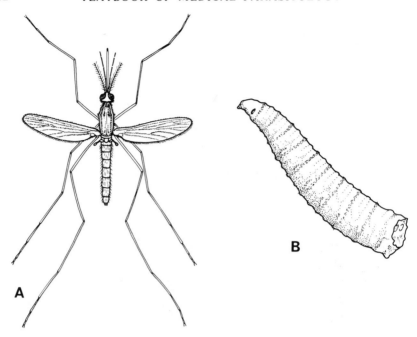

FIG. 9. (A) *Anopheles,* a mosquito dipteran; (B) a fly maggot.

is secondarily infected or there are allergic reactions connected with the bite. In such an event, diagnosis of what kind of insect bite is involved is of minor practical importance in comparison to the symptomatic treatment of the patient. All dipterans have a single pair of functional, membranous wings (Fig. 9A), and there are various modifications of their mouthparts. Such dipterans as mosquitoes and deer flies have piercing and sucking mouthparts; the house fly sops up fluid by fleshy pads located at the end of its proboscis; and the horse fly makes a wound in the integument by cutting stylets and then sops up blood.

Treatment. Palliative lotions and antiseptic measures are usually all that are required.

Post-Treatment Advice. Patients who are particularly sensitive should be advised as to the value of various insect repellants.

SELECTED REFERENCES

Arean, V. M., and Fox, I. 1955. Dermal alterations in severe reactions to bite of the sandfly, *Culicoides furens. J. Clin. Pathol., 25:* 1359.

Bates, M. 1949. *The Natural History of Mosquitoes.* 379 pp., Macmillan Company, New York.

Smart, J. 1956. *A Handbook for the Identification of Insects of Medical Importance.* 363 pp., British Museum, London.

MYIASIS

Various fly larvae

Myiasis denotes various degrees of infection in a patient with the larvae or maggots of various flies. The association may be one in which the insect larva requires living tissue for its development and metamorphosis; where the maggot may develop either in living or nonliving organic matter; or cases in which maggots are incidentally ingested, and the human gut otherwise plays no regular role in the development of the insect. The flies whose larvae may be involved in a myiasis case include bot flies, warble flies, screw worms, blow flies, flesh flies, bottle flies and latrine flies.

Clinical Picture. The different possibilities of clinical involvement are numerous and depend mostly on the area of the body involved and the kind and number of maggots involved. In those larvae involving the integument, there is usually a painful, nonprogressing ulcer or raised serpiginous tunnels in the skin, accompanied by swelling and fever in the patient. In some cases the larvae proceed to deep tissue (even the brain), and the symptomatology in such cases depends on what part of the body is involved. Atrial openings, such as the nares, mouth, ear, and the genitourinary tract, may also be infected with various fly larvae. In the case of intestinal myiasis, nausea and diarrhea are frequent aspects of the infection.

Life Cycle. Infection with fly larvae is circumstantial, and the association may be obligate, facultative or accidental. The larvae of some fly species are deposited directly into wounds or skin abrasions, whereas in other species the female fly deposits eggs or even larvae on human skin. Some species utilize other flies in transmission whereby eggs are deposited on the body of a blood-sucking arthropod and transported to human skin at the time of a blood meal. These eggs then hatch and penetrate the human integument and later reside or migrate to various deeper body tissues.

Diagnosis. Definite diagnosis can be made only on identification of the fly maggot—which is worm-like, segmented and pointed anteriorly (Fig. 9B). The blunt posterior end has a pair of stigmal plates which bear respiratory pores. Since morphology of these plates is of diagnostic value in determining the type of insect involved, an entomologist or parasitologist should be consulted for specific diagnosis. Myiasis-producing insects are widely distributed in nature and involve man and many other animals.

Treatment. Surgical and antiseptic measures are required in cutaneous and other tissue infections, whereas in intestinal myiasis vari-

ous purgatives are indicated. Urinary myiasis is usually self-termi-
nating.

Post-Treatment Advice. Prevention is the keynote in myiasis cases.
Measures of value for patients who run a high risk include insecticiding
breeding places of the flies, the use of insect repellants, and the proper
care in food preparation and wound management.

SELECTED REFERENCES

Dalmat, H. T. 1955. Cutaneous myiasis of the scalp due to *Dermatobia hominis. Amer. J.
Trop. Med. & Hyg., 4:* 334.
James, M. T. 1947. The flies that cause myiasis in man. *U. S. Dept. Agric. Misc. Publ.
No. 631,* 172 pp., Washington, D. C.
Stabler, R. M., Nelson, M. C., Lewis, B. J., and Berthong, M. 1962. *Wohlfartia opaca*
myiasis in man in Colorado. *J. Parasitol., 28:* 249.

CUTANEOUS LEISHMANIASIS

Oriental sore   *Leishmania tropica*

Clinical Picture. Protozoan flagellates are responsible for cutaneous
leishmaniasis, or Oriental sore, in a patient. A papule first forms at
the site of a bite from an infected sandfly. This lesion then develops
into a shallow sore with raised edges. It then goes on to ulcerate, but
pus is not formed unless the sore is secondarily infected. The sore
eventually ends up as a disfiguring, depressed, depigmented scar. There
may be several sores on a patient due to several insect bites. The parasites in the reticuloendothelial cells pack at the base and edges of the
sore and may extend to neighboring lymph nodes but do not invade
the viscera. Based on clinical, immunologic and epidemiologic grounds,
there are two kinds of cutaneous leishmaniasis—the *dry type* and the
wet type.

The dry type is an urban disease, has a long incubation period and
late ulceration, exhibits numerous parasites in the lesions, and does
not very often involve lymph nodes.

The wet type is a rural disease, has a short incubation period and
ulcerates early, shows scanty parasites in the lesion, and more often
involves neighboring lymph nodes.

Life Cycle. Whether the disease is of the dry or wet type, it is still
transmitted by the female sandfly. The infective parasites which are
introduced into the skin of a patient by the insect bite are flagellated
leptomonal organisms. These parasites round up and assume the
leishmanial form of the parasite in macrophages and other reticuloendothelial cells of subcutaneous tissues. The incubation period may
vary from a week to several months. The leishmanial organisms mul-

tiply in the RE cells until the latter rupture, after which the parasitic progeny repeat the cycle in other suitable cells. Whereas the dry type of the disease is mostly a man-to-man transmission, the wet type is primarily an infection of rodents and dogs.

Diagnosis. Any cutaneous ulcer on a patient who has resided in an endemic area is suspect of leishmaniasis. Since the gross lesion may resemble lesions of blastomycosis and other infections, the only certainty of diagnosis is the microscopic identification of the leishmanial parasites. A smear is taken from the edges and base of the sore and stained with Giemsa's or Wright's stain. If the parasites are present, they can be seen either in RE cells or free in the smear preparation.

The leishmanial organisms are oval bodies, measuring about 2 μ in diameter and containing a distinct nucleus and much smaller kinetoplast (Fig. 10A). Culture is also possible on blood agar, and laboratory rodents are susceptible to experimental infection. The morphologic form of the parasite in culture would be the leptomonal form (Fig. 10B), whereas in rodents the leishmanial parasites can be demonstrated from macrophages, especially of the spleen and liver. Cutaneous leishmaniasis occurs mostly in the Middle East, Asia, and the Mediterranean area, although there have been reports of it also in Latin America.

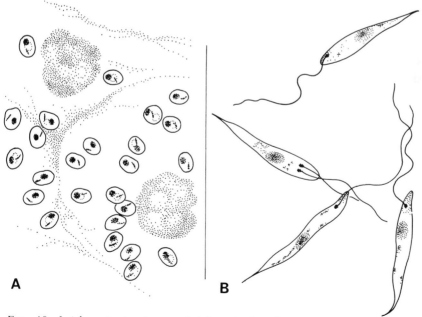

A   **B**

FIG. 10. *Leishmania tropica* or *Leishmania braziliensis*: (A) Portions of two macrophages containing leishmanial forms of the parasite; (B) leptomonal forms from culture.

Treatment. If a patient is to remain in an endemic area, the sore probably should be allowed to self-terminate, since there is complete immunity to subsequent infection (although there is no cross immunity between the dry and wet types). If the patient is to remain outside an endemic area, then antibiotics are administered for possible secondary infection, and either quinacrine or trivalent antimony (such as stibophen) is injected at the sore site for action against the flagellates. Multiple or advanced lesions should be treated systemically with ethylstibamine.

Post-Treatment Advice. Active and complete immunity of a patient may be effected by inoculating living parasites into an area of the skin of little cosmetic value. The residual spraying of households with DDT is effective in controlling sandflies.

SELECTED REFERENCES

Kurban, A. K. 1966. Histopathology of cutaneous leishmaniasis. *Arch. Dermatol., 93:* 396.

Manson-Bahr, P. E. C. 1964. Variations in the clinical manifestations of leishmaniasis caused by *L. tropica. J. Trop. Med., 67:* 85.

AMERICAN CUTANEOUS LEISHMANIASIS

Espundia

Chiclero ulcer } *Leishmania braziliensis*

Uta ulcer

Clinical Picture. American cutaneous leishmaniasis exists in Latin America as several clinical types. These are probably based on strain differences of the parasitic flagellates that are responsible for the disease. The early course is similar to Oriental sore—a papule forms at the site of the sandfly bite and transforms into a pustule which then ulcerates. In the Mexican "chiclero" and South American "uta" types the lesions rarely metastasize to other areas of the body. The chiclero ulcer is usually confined to the ears, whereas the uta type resembles Oriental sore and may be located anywhere on the exposed part of the body. In the classical "espundia" mucocutaneous type of South America there is secondary spread of the initial lesion to mucocutaneous junctions, especially the nose, throat and buccal area. The espundia type of leishmaniasis may be most mutilating, in which there is extensive multiplication of the leishmanial parasites, and erosion and destruction of cartilage and bone. In this type secondary microbial infection plays a considerable role in the course of the disease. There also seem to be several intermediate clinical types of American cutaneous leishmaniasis.

Life Cycle. The life cycle of the parasitic organisms of American cutaneous leishmaniasis resembles that of Oriental sore. The chief distinction is the relative invasiveness of the parasite and the subsequent course of the disease. A number of sylvatic rodents are known to act as chief hosts of various strains of the parasite, and in some cases dogs are involved as reservoir hosts.

Diagnosis. The lesions of some forms of American cutaneous leishmaniasis may be confused with those of blastomycosis, yaws, leprosy and other infections. As in all leishmaniasis cases diagnosis depends mostly on microscopic identification of the *leishmanial* parasites (Fig. 10A) from smears of the involved areas. The organisms are morphologically identical to those of Oriental sore. Culture (Fig. 10B) is possible on blood agar, especially in the early stages of the disease. In late infections both microscopic identification and culture of the organisms are difficult, especially if the lesion(s) are complicated by bacterial invasion. An intracutaneous skin test (using whole or fractionated antigen of cultured organisms) is useful in diagnosis. Positive reactions are of the delayed type, and false positives have been reported. The various types of the disease are distributed throughout Latin America.

Treatment. There does not seem to be any lasting immunity after American cutaneous leishmaniasis cases, as there is in Oriental sore. Antibiotics are used for secondary infections, and there is a variety of drugs that have been used against the parasites. Trivalent antimonials (such as stibophen) are useful for early lesions, but some cases have responded better to arsenical treatment (such as Neosalvarsan). The pentavalent antimonial, ethylstibamine, has been very useful in arresting the spread of infections to other body sites. In patients resistant to antimonials, such drugs as pentamidine, pyrimethamine and amphotericin B, have proved effective.

Post-Treatment Advice. Residual spraying of households with DDT is of value in the control of sandflies. Insect repellants are useful to patients who are forest or field workers.

SELECTED REFERENCES

Convit, J., and Kerdel-Vegas, F. 1965. Disseminated cutaneous leishmaniasis. *Arch. Dermatol., 91:* 439.
Omran, Abdel-Rahim. 1961. The ecology of leishmaniasis. IN *Studies in Disease Ecology,* J. M. May, Ed., pp. 331–388, Hafner Publishing Company, Inc., New York.

SCHISTOSOME DERMATITIS

Swimmer's itch   Various bird and mammalian cercariae

Clinical Picture. A patient with swimmer's itch, or schistosome dermatitis, develops a rash soon after contact with fresh water environ-

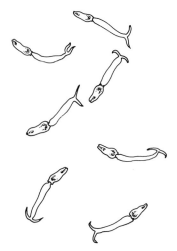

FIG. 11. Cercarial larvae of schistosomes.

ments or some marine beaches. The skin exhibits petechial hemorrhages, papular eruptions, intense itching, and some edema. There is
an allergic basis for this integumentary condition so that sensitive patients develop more severe reactions in multiple exposures to the
trematode parasite. Urticaria may develop in these patients, and the
intense itching and scratching may lead to secondary infection of the
original skin lesions.

Life Cycle. Swimmer's itch is acquired when a patient's skin comes
into contact with the free-living larval form of nonhuman blood flukes.
The species involved are normally parasites of water birds and also
some smaller feral animals. These *cercarial larvae* (Fig. 11) penetrate
human skin but do not produce a permanent infection, being walled off
in the epithelial layers of the skin. It is a blind alley infection, and the
larvae soon die and are absorbed.

Diagnosis. Diagnosis is based on signs and symptoms after leaving
the aquatic environment.

Treatment. Palliative lotions, such as calamine, are all that are indicated, except that antihistamines may be required in severe cases, and
antimicrobials when secondary infection is present.

Post-Treatment Advice. Since most cercarial penetration takes place
when the water evaporates from the patient's skin, brisk rubbing with
a towel after leaving the water reduces greatly the number of larvae
which penetrate. Such a practice should be suggested to patients who
run a high risk of schistosome dermatitis because of occupational or
recreational habits. Treating the shore line of fresh-water environments

with copper sulfate is a fairly effective measure in controlling the snails which release the cercarial organisms into the water.

SELECTED REFERENCES

Hunter, G. W., III. 1960. Studies on schistosomiasis. XIII. Schistosome dermatitis in Colorado. *J. Parasitol.*, *46:* 231.
Olivier, L. 1949. Schistosome dermatitis, a sensitization reaction. *Amer. J. Hyg.*, *49:* 209.
Stauber, L. A. 1958. Swimmer's itch in New Jersey. *J. Parasitol.*, *44:* 108.

SPARGANOSIS

Plerocercoid tapeworm larvae   *Spirometra*

Clinical Picture. The effects of human infection with plerocercoid, or spargana, tapeworm larvae vary according to the location of the parasites in the body. The larvae migrate in subcutaneous tissues and muscles and elicit inflammatory reactions but no fibrotic encapsulation. There may be chills, fever and general discomfort in the patient, and the larvae may be very painful and cause intense itching and pressure symptoms. Those larvae which cease migrating appear as subcutaneous nodules or tumors. In cases where the eye is involved, there may be painful periorbital edema. Some spargana larvae break up in the body, and the pieces develop individually. This miliary situation is very serious.

Life Cycle. A patient becomes infected by interposing in the usual life cycle of the tapeworm. The adult worms live in the intestine of dogs and cats, and the first intermediate host requires a crustacean copepod. The tapeworm eggs are released in the feces of the infected dog or cat, and after suitable incubation in water, ciliated embryos hatch out and swim in the water. Copepods eat these organisms, and within the crustacean body there develops a larva called the procercoid. When infected copepods are ingested by a variety of animals (frogs, tadpoles, snakes, birds), there develops in these animals another type of larva called the *plerocercoid* or *sparganum*. Cats or dogs eating animals with the infective sparganum larva soon develop adult tapeworms in their intestines. Man happens to be an unsuitable host for the development of the sparganum larva to an adult worm; therefore, his acquiring the infection results in no further development beyond that stage.

A patient may become infected by drinking water containing copepods infected with the procercoid stage of the worm. In such cases the procercoids penetrate the human intestine and eventually end up in subcutaneous tissues as spargana larvae.

In some areas of the world where snakes and frogs are a common item in the diet, these infected animals serve as a source of human infection. In countries where frog and tadpole meat poultices are applied to sore eyes or open lesions, the spargana from such infected meat can be transferred to a patient, resulting in either ocular or subcutaneous sparganosis.

The geographic distribution of human sparganosis is world-wide but especially prevalent in the Far East. There have been several species reported from man, but on practical grounds they can be all grouped together as simply sparganum cases.

Diagnosis. The only method of diagnosis is by identification of the sparganum larva in biopsied material. Any subcutaneous nodule should suggest sparganosis, especially if there is history of its appearing and disappearing. Some workers have suggested that many subcutaneous lipomas may be sparganum infections; therefore, in the microscopic examinations of sections of such tumors consideration should be made of tapeworm larvae. The sparganum larva is whitish, wrinkled, grossly visible to the unaided eye, and has two grooved-out areas at one end (Fig. 12). Its identification in sections requires knowledge of tapeworm morphology.

Treatment. Surgical removal of the larva is the only means of treatment, but this may be quite difficult in the case of ocular sparganosis.

Post-Treatment Advice. The potential danger of drinking non-

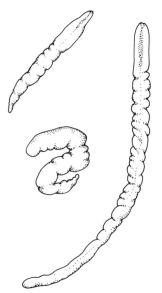

Fig. 12. Spargana tapeworm larvae: three parasites excised from subcutaneous tissue.

municipal water and the practice of applying snake or amphibian poultices to the eyes or skin should be pointed out.

SELECTED REFERENCES

Cross, J. H. 1963. Sparganosis in two members of an Arkansas family. *J. Parasitol., 49:* 154.

Markell, E. K., and Haber, S. L. 1963. A case of human sparganosis from California. *Amer. J. Med., 37:* 491.

Mueller, J. F., Hart, E. P., and Walsh, W. A. 1963. Human sparganosis in the United States. *J. Parasitol., 49:* 294.

Read, C. P. 1952. Human sparganosis in south Texas. *J. Parasitol., 38:* 29.

CUTANEOUS LARVA MIGRANS

Creeping eruption   *Ancylostoma braziliense*

Clinical Picture. Creeping eruption, or cutaneous larva migrans, of a patient is characterized initially by red, itchy papules in the area of the involved skin. In a few days, these sites become erythemic and develop into advancing, serpiginous, raised tunnels. There is uncontrollable itching, and scratching often leads to secondary infection. The posterior end of the tunnel becomes crusty, and the tunnels may advance several millimeters per day. In extreme cases the lesions may cover a large area of the skin, but usually they are confined only to

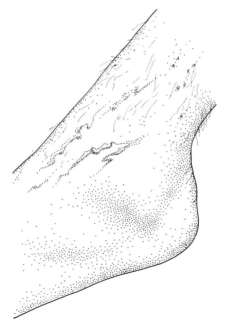

Fig. 13. Creeping eruption lesions on ankle region. (Based on photograph in Brook's *Essentials of Medical Parasitology,* The Macmillan Co., New York).

the hands and feet. Some patients have exhibited systemic reactions.

Life Cycle. A patient acquires the infection by coming into contact with skin-penetrating hookworms which normally inhabit cats and dogs. The papules develop around the initial penetration sites, and the cutaneous tunnels represent the wandering worm larvae in the layers of the skin. Most of the larvae are destroyed by cellular infiltration, but some may persist for several weeks. In cats and dogs these same larvae would eventually reach and mature in the small intestine. Worm eggs are released in the feces of infected cats and dogs, hatch and eventually develop into skin-penetrating larvae in the soil.

Diagnosis. Gross observations of the lesions and advancing tunnels (Fig. 13) is usually sufficient for diagnosis, but these have some resemblance to some fly larvae infections of human skin and other cutaneous lesions caused by skin penetration of other nematodes. Creeping eruption is found anywhere that patients come into contact with soil contaminated with cat and dog feces.

Treatment. Palliative lotions are indicated and antihistamines in sensitive cases. Some cases terminate without treatment, but others may persist for several weeks. Thiabendazole has been reported to be a highly curative chemotherapeutic agent but has not been approved as yet as a human drug.

Post-Treatment Advice. Most cases involve children, who have a higher rate of contact with soil. Various occupations of adults also place them in a high risk category. Advice for prevention includes periodic de-worming of cat and dog pets and the covering of children's sand boxes when not in use.

SELECTED REFERENCES

Stone, O. J., and Mullins, J. F. 1964. Thiabendazole therapy for creeping eruption. *Arch. Dermatol., 89:* 557.

Katz, R., Ziegler, J., and Blank, H. 1965. The natural course of creeping eruption and treatment with thiabendazole. *Arch. Dermatol., 91:* 420.

DRACUNCULIASIS

Guinea worm   *Dracunculus medinensis*

Clinical Picture. When the female Guinea worm nematode is in the connective tissue areas of deeper parts of the body, there are little or no symptoms in an infected patient. It is when the worm makes its way to the skin surface that signs and symptoms develop. General allergic reactions—such as urticaria and eosinophilia, vomiting, giddiness, and burning and itching sensations—may occur. A blister then develops on the skin (usually the lower extremities), which then goes on to ulcerate. Even though the blister is initially sterile, it usually becomes infected with bacteria, and the sore ulcerates and develops moderate to severe necrosis. The allergic reactions ordinarily cease after the development of the blister and ulcer.

Life Cycle. A patient becomes infected by ingesting (in drinking water) copepods infected with the larval stage of the parasite. These larvae penetrate the human small intestine and mature in the subcutaneous and deeper connective tissue areas of the body after several months. The role of the pigmy-sized male worms is poorly known. The female worm may attain a length of about a meter at maturity (when she migrates to the skin surface).

At the time of blister formation on human skin, the female worm is almost exclusively a container of larval embryos. A piece of her uterus then prolapses either through her mouth or through a break in the anterior body wall, and the larvae are released into the lesion when it comes into contact with water. The worm uterus heals over when the infected lesion dries out, so that there is a successive release of larvae each time the patient's lesion makes contact with water. When suitable copepod crustaceans eat the active nematode larvae, there is further development of the parasite in the copepod for several weeks.

Guinea worm infection is widely distributed in Africa, the Middle and Far East, and certain parts of the Americas. There are several feral animals which also harbor the infection, and there is also a closely related species of this worm in wild animals.

Diagnosis. There is no method of diagnosing the infection in the early phase. The skin lesion (Fig. 14) is the point of diagnostic importance. The uterus may be seen protruding from the sore, or, if not, the lesion is bathed in cold water and the water examined microscopically for the nematode larvae.

Treatment. The ancient practice of enticing the worm to come out by successive douches and then winding it a little at a time on a stick is still used. Such extraction may take up to two weeks to get the worm out. If the nematode breaks, severe secondary infection usually results; hence, this practice is to be used with caution. If one has enough patience, the worm can be continuously "milked" by douching, after which it is usually resorbed or expelled with little or no difficulty.

Phenothiazine injected close to the worm apparently kills it, or at least permits easier extraction or quicker absorption in case it breaks. Diethylcarbamazine (Hetrazan) is lethal to the immature worm, but since diagnosis cannot be made in the early stages, it has had little

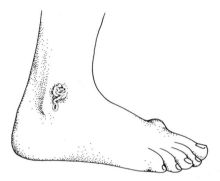

FIG. 14. Lesions of dracunculiasis on foot: uterus of worm protruding from ankle region; another non-erupted lesion in profile. (Based on photograph in Markell & Voge's *Medical Parasitology*, W. B. Saunders Co., Philadelphia).

practical use (unless there are additional unsurfaced worms in the patient). Corticosteroids and antihistamines are used for allergic reactions, and antibiotics are in order in the case of secondary bacterial infections.

Post-Treatment Advice. Since water sources are what they are in endemic areas, there is little practical advice one can give a patient tied to these conditions.

SELECTED REFERENCE

Hodgson, C., and Barrett, D. F. 1964. Chronic dracunculosis. *Brit. J. Dermatol.*, *76*: 211.

ONCHOCERCIASIS

River blindness   *Onchocerca volvulus*

Clinical Picture. Onchocerciasis is caused by a filarial nematode which is found almost exclusively in tissue and not in the vascular system, as is true with other filarial worms. The adults locate subcutaneously in tangled knots and are encapsulated by fibrous tissue. The subcutaneous nodules so characteristic of this infection are located chiefly on the scalp and shoulders of patients from Central America, whereas in Africa the trunk region of the body is more frequently involved. The female worms lay active, microscopic embryos (microfilariae), which escape encapsulation and may locate in any portion of the integument. During this period there are considerable allergic reactions in the patient. The nodules may be quite painful, and considerable eosinophilia is the rule.

The most serious aspect of onchocerciasis involves the eye. The microfilariae enter various portions of the eye, and in infections of long duration, there develops photophobia, visual impairment, and blindness due to retinal and optic nerve damage.

Life Cycle. The infection is transmitted by the black fly or buffalo gnat. This insect introduces infective larvae with its bite, and these migrate in the skin of a patient and eventually mature into male and female worms in several months. Vascular infiltration and eventual fibrosis sets in around the worms, later developing into a tough, fibrous nodule. As mentioned, the microfilariae are released by the female nematodes, and they move throughout the cutaneous areas. When microfilariae from an infective patient are sucked up by a black fly, they undergo further development in the insect and eventually migrate to the proboscis and are infective when introduced into human skin. Although there are related species in other animals, there do not seem to be any reservoirs of infection to this human pathogen.

Diagnosis. Although adult worms can be identified from surgical removal of nodules (Fig. 15B, 15C), the simplest diagnostic technique is by examining skin scrapings or shavings in which the microfilariae can be microscopically identified. The microfilariae *lack* a sheath around the cylindrical body of the parasite (Fig. 15A).

Treatment. The most accepted course of action is a combination of

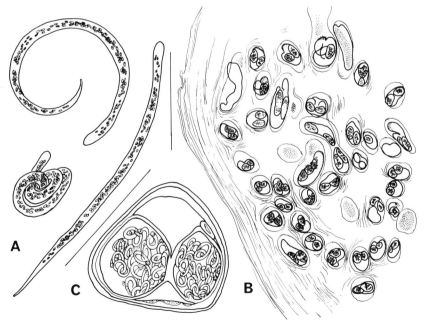

FIG. 15. *Onchocerca volvulus*: (A) three non-sheathed microfilariae from skin scraping; (B) Section through skin nodule, showing many worms; (C) enlargement of a section, showing microfilariae in uterus.

surgical removal of the subcutaneous nodules and chemotherapy. Removal of all visible nodules is important in the prevention of eye damage. Diethylcarbamazine (Hetrazan) is active against the microfilariae, and suramin (Bayer 205) kills the adult worms. It should be emphasized that the killing of microfilariae may result in severe allergic reactions, so the use of Hetrazan may require the concomitant use of corticosteroids or antihistamines. Since allergic reactions also affect the eye, the use of Hetrazan alone may actually increase eye damage.

Post-Treatment Advice. There is little practical advice one can give regarding prevention of infection. Following treatment, any further nodular development should be excised at an early date.

SELECTED REFERENCES

Burch, T. A. 1961. The ecology of onchocerciasis. IN *Studies in Disease Ecology.* J. M. May, Ed. pp. 73–88, Hafner Publishing Company, New York.
Woodruff, A. W., Bell, S., Ridley, D. S., and Schofield, F. D. 1958. Clinical, diagnostic, and therapeutic aspects of onchocercosis. *Trans. Roy. Soc. Trop. Med. & Hyg., 52:* 97.
——, Barnley, G. R., Holland, J. T., Jones, D. E., McCrae, A. W. R., and McLaren, D. S. 1963. Onchocerciasis and the eye in western Uganda. *Trans. Roy. Soc. Trop. Med. & Hyg., 57:* 50.

ARACHNIDISM

Black widow spider   *Latrodectus mactans*

Clinical Picture. The effect of black widow spider bite is due to a potent peripheral neurotoxin injected with the bite. As is true with all cases of venomous animals, the clinical picture depends on such factors as the amount of venom injected, and the age, weight and sensitivity of the patient. The venom in spiders is released from a pair of jaw-like structures so a patient shows a small pair of puncture wounds in aposition, usually on the genitalia, buttocks or extremities.

A few minutes after the bite there is sharp pain but little or no swelling. This is followed by reddening, swelling and burning of the bite area. Relatively, the toxin is absorbed quickly and distributed by the vascular system, after which systemic reactions ensue. These include numbness, ascending paralysis, abdominal tetanic cramps (highly characteristic), shallow respiration, hyperarterial pressure, and convulsions. Shock may result and death due to respiratory failure. In recovered cases there may be peripheral numbness for several days.

Life Cycle. Black widow spider contact may occur either in or outside of the household, and as in all venomous animal bites, a bitten patient should be considered a toxicologic case. It is the female spider alone that is dangerous, as the small, feeble male delivers an ineffective bite, plus the fact that he is usually eaten by the female after copulation (a practice highly developed in spiders). Other aspects of the life cycle have little clinical significance.

Diagnosis. If the patient was aware of being bitten by the black widow spider, diagnosis presents no problems. If he was not aware or was uncertain, then the systemic clinical picture (when the bite marks can be discerned) is sufficient for diagnosis. Since the bite marks on the genitalia and buttocks may be overlooked and since the general symptomatology resembles peritonitis, tetanus and perforated ulcer, there have been cases in which needless emergency operations have been performed. The morphologic characteristics of the female black widow spider are: 4 pairs of long, hairy legs, a small cephalothorax connected by a very thin waist to a large, rounded, unsegmented abdomen; and the spider is black with orange or red markings on the ventral surface, often in the form of hour-glass figures (Fig. 16). There may also be colored markings on the dorsal side. This spider is found both in the New and Old World.

Treatment. If less than 30 minutes has passed and the patient has a bite on an extremity, a proximal tourniquet should be applied as soon as possible and incision and suction administered as in snakebite. Cryotherapy is effective before systemic reactions commence. Intra-

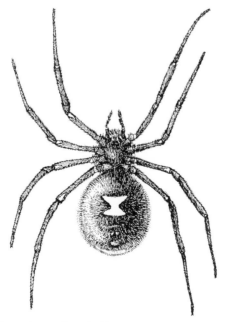

FIG. 16. *Latrodectus*, female black widow spider, ventral view.

venous calcium gluconate relieves tetanic contractions, and corticoster-oids sometimes give rapid relief. Hot baths and packs are effective in producing vasodilation in a critical case. Intramuscular antivenin is available, and if used, the patient should be tested to the horse serum vehicle and desensitized if necessary.

Post-Treatment Advice. DDT spraying of privies or the household is effective in controlling spiders.

SELECTED REFERENCES

Horen, W. P. 1963. Arachnidism in the United States. *J.A.M.A., 185:* 839.

Maretic, Z., and Stanic, M. 1954. The health problem of arachnidism. *Bull. Wld. Hlth. Org., 11:* 1007.

Peters, L. E. 1962. Black widow spider bite. *Texas State J. Med., 58:* 87.

NECROTIC ARACHNIDISM

Brown spider   *Loxosceles*

Clinical Picture. Although the effects of hemolytic substances have been recorded in some cases of brown spider bite, the chief results have to do with a necrotizing toxin. As is true with most animal toxins, this one is a combination of pharmacologically active fractions, and the clinical picture in a patient depends on the amount and potency of the toxin and the age and sensitivity of the patient. The usual case involves only a slightly painful bite at first, followed by pain, swelling and bleb formation at the bite site. The bleb then sloughs and may be followed by radiating necrosis and deep ulceration. After about a week there develops a black scab over the ulcer. The whole lesion takes weeks or months to heal, and plastic surgery may be required as an aftermath. If hemolysin is involved, there may be systemic reactions—such as hematuria—and, in fatal cases, cardiac failure.

Life Cycle. Since the brown spider is largely a domestic species, bites are usually acquired inside the household or in other buildings. As with black widow spider bite, it is the female spider that is important in necrotic arachnidism. Various species of the brown spider are distributed in Latin America but also occur in various parts of North America.

Diagnosis. Bleb formation around puncture marks and the nature of the developing lesion are sufficient to establish diagnosis. The face and upper extremities are more often bitten than the lower parts of the body. If the spider is brought in by a patient, it can be easily identified. In addition to being a medium-sized, fawn-colored spider, it has a characteristic glossy, violin-shaped decoration on its cephalothorax (Fig. 17).

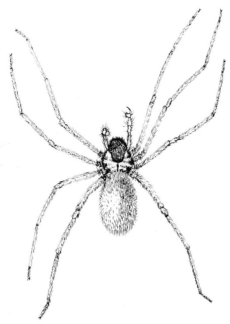

FIG. 17. *Loxoceles*, female brown spider, dorsal view.

Treatment. Since antivenin is currently unavailable, corticosteroids should be administered as early as possible as an antihemolytic measure and to hasten the healing time of the lesion. Otherwise, all other measures are empirical in terms of the cutaneous lesion.

Post-Treatment Advice. DDT spraying of the house, particularly closets, is effective in controlling spiders.

SELECTED REFERENCES

Atkins, J. A., Wingo, G. W., Sodeman, W. A., and Flynn, J. E. 1958. Necrotic arachnidism. *Amer. J. Trop. Med. & Hyg., 7:* 165.

Blattner, R. J. 1958. Necrotic arachnidism. *J. Pediatr., 53:* 377.

Minton, S. A., Jr., and Olson, C. 1964. A case of spider bite with severe hemolytic reaction. *Pediatrics, 33:* 283.

SCORPIONS

Centruroides

Clinical Picture. The effect of scorpion sting in a patient is protean and varies according to such factors as the species and age of the scorpion, the kind and amount of venom injected, and the age, weight and sensitivity of the patient. Although some venoms cause little or no damage to the body, others may be quite serious. In most venoms of scorpions there are neurotoxic, hemorrhagic and hemolytic fractions. A stung patient usually has a single puncture wound, mostly on the arm or leg.

If the amount of neurotoxin is small or lacking, there will be little or no systemic effects but rather local reactions around the sting wound. These include sharp pains, swelling, and lymph node enlargement in the affected area. The patient usually feels better in several hours.

In scorpion stings which have relatively more neurotoxin, there is a minimal local reaction but rather severe systemic effects. Sharp, itching pains are followed by muscle twitching, vomiting, convulsions, profuse salivation, thirst—and, in fatal cases, edema of the lungs, cyanosis, and respiratory paralysis.

Life Cycle. A patient's contact with scorpions is accidental and may occur either inside or outside the household. Scorpions are nocturnal in habit, and during the day they rest under logs, rocks and other dark, moist places. It is also during this period that they migrate into the household. Both male and female scorpions can sting, although the young and smaller-sized species are unable to penetrate the human integument. Though poisonous scorpions are found in many areas of the world, those of medical importance in North America are confined mostly to Mexico and the southwestern part of the United States.

Diagnosis. Local or systemic signs and symptoms are usually suffi-

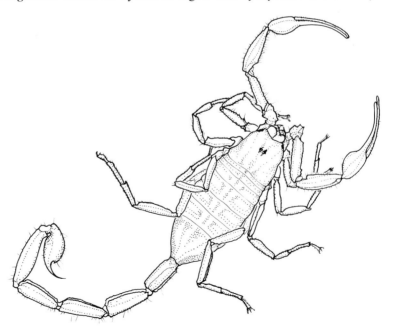

FIG. 18. *Centruroides* scorpion.

cient to establish diagnosis, especially if the patient observed or brought in the scorpion. These animals have an elongate, segmented abdomen, the tip of which has a stinger. The abdomen is flexed forward during the striking procedure, and the venom is ejected from the abdominal stinger. In addition to 4 pairs of legs, scorpions also have a large pair of crab-like pincers at the anterior end of the body (Fig. 18). There are other nonpoisonous arachnids that strongly resemble scorpions; therefore, if there is a taxonomic question in a given case, an entomologist or parasitologist should be consulted.

Treatment. If there is severe local reaction but no systemic symptoms, palliative treatment is all that is necessary. If there is little or no reaction around the sting and a poisonous species has been established, a tourniquet should be applied proximal to the wound as quickly as possible. Pain may be relieved by analgesics and local spraying with ethyl chloride. Antivenom can be obtained from the Poisonous Animals Research Laboratory, Tempe, Arizona, and is effective if administered soon after the sting. Measures should be taken to combat shock. Very young children with systemic symptoms should be considered as medical emergencies.

Post-Treatment Advice. There is little practical advice one can give, except that Chlordane or Lindane house spraying is effective in controlling scorpions.

SELECTED REFERENCES

Potter, J. M., and Northey, W. T. 1962. Immunological evaluation of scorpion venoms. *Amer. J. Trop. Med. & Hyg., 11:* 712.

Stahnke, H. L. 1961. *Scorpions* (Pamphlet). Poisonous Animals Research Laboratory, Arizona State University, Tempe, Arizona.

WASPS AND BEES

Clinical Picture. The effects of wasp or bee sting depend on the nature and amount of toxin introduced and the hypersensitivity of the patient. Although most patients experience nothing more than local pain, edema, and wheal and flare at the point of the sting, others are affected violently and often fatally. Bee and wasp venom is a multifactor toxin, and its constituents include hemolytic, neurotoxic, histamine-like, decreased coagulative, and hyaluronidase fractions. The degree of hypersensitivity in a patient determines the seriousness of a case. In severe cases there is pronounced pain and swelling, urticaria, vomiting, asthmatic attacks leading to convulsions, and respiratory and cardiac failures.

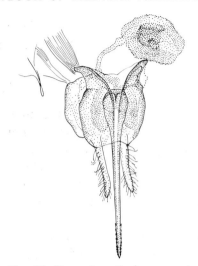

FIG. 19. Honey bee stinging apparatus.

Life Cycle. Bee and wasp sting in a patient is an accidental circumstance, and the life cycle of these arthropods has no clinical significance. The potential seriousness is a consequence of the allergic response of a stung patient to toxin, although some feel that allergy may also be connected with the pollen that these arthropods invariably carry.

Diagnosis. A patient is usually aware that he has been stung by a wasp or bee. The stinger is located at the hind end of these insects. Honey bees and some wasps sting only once (the stinger almost always is left in the patient's skin), whereas the stinger of bumble bees and most wasps is not released, and these insects can sting over and over again. When there is some question as to what stung a patient, the presence of a stinger is helpful in diagnosis (Fig. 19).

Treatment. If the stinger is in the skin, the first step should be to carefully remove it, so as not to squeeze more toxin into the integument. This is accomplished by teasing the stinger out with a needle or sharp blade. The lesion should be treated with palliative and bacteriostatic ointments. If the patient is known to be hypersensitive, if there are multiple stings, or if the pain and swelling are severe and there are indications of systemic symptoms, the case should be considered a medical emergency.

If the wound is on the extremities, a proximal tourniquet should be applied. Cryotherapy, if applied early enough, will alleviate pain and swelling (as will local injection of antihistamines) and reduce the rate of toxin absorption. If anaphylactoid signs are apparent, epinephrine or ethyl norepinephrine should be administered (intravenous if necessary).

Post-Treatment Advice. Patients known or found to be sensitive to bee or wasp sting should be encouraged to always carry on their person an emergency kit having the necessary materials for self-treatment. Such patients should also be instructed in the use of such a kit. In patients with extreme hypersensitivity, the wearing of allergy identification (in the form of a locket, bracelet or dog tags) should be encouraged. Such patients should also be encouraged to undergo a desensitization program with group antigens of wasps and bees.

SELECTED REFERENCES

Brown, H. 1963. Allergy to certain hymenoptera: bees, hornets, wasps, and yellow jackets. *J.A.M.A., 18:* 137.

Frazier, C. A. 1964. Allergic reactions to insect stings: A review of 180 cases. *Southern Med. J., 57:* 1028.

—— 1965. Insect sting reactions in children. *Ann. Allergy, 23:* 37.

Parrish, H. M. 1963. Analysis of 460 fatalities from venomous animals in the United States. *Amer. J. Med. Sci., 245:* 129.

Shaffer, J. H. 1961. Stinging insects—a treat of life. *J.A.M.A., 177:* 473.

FIRE ANT

Solenopsis

Clinical Picture. Although patient contact with most ants produces only relatively minor effects which can be easily controlled, the sting of fire ants can be quite serious. The venom of this insect has both hemolytic and necrotizing properties. These ants do not lose their stinger, so there may be several sting marks on the patient's skin. A flare and wheal develops around the puncture, followed by bleb formation which may then go on to ulceration. During the early phases of the lesion there is extreme pain and intense itching in the patient. The lesion may become necrotic and heal very slowly (as in brown spider bite), and scar formation may be rather extensive. Some patients are hypersensitive to the sting and exhibit fever and anaphylactoid shock.

Life Cycle. Contact with the fire ant is accidental, and the seriousness of the sting relates mostly to the allergic response of the patient.

Diagnosis. The skin lesion is characteristic, and the ant is usually brought in for identification. Fire ants are distributed in the southeastern section of the United States.

Treatment. Cryotherapy and palliative lotions are used for local effects, whereas antihistamines and epinephrine are in order for shock.

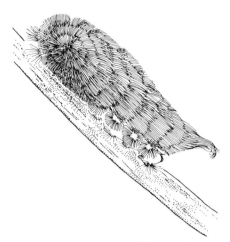

FIG. 20. Puss caterpillar on twig.

Post-Treatment Advice. Lawns may be treated with chemicals as an anti-ant control measure. Contact with ant mounds should be avoided.

SELECTED REFERENCES

Adrouny, G. A., Derbes, V. J., and Jung, R. C. 1959. Isolation of a hemolytic component of fire ant venom. *Science, 130:* 449.

Caro, M. R., Derbes, V. J., and Jung, R. C. 1957. Skin responses to the sting of the imported fire ant (*Solenopsis saevissima*). *Arch. Dermatol. Syphilol., 75:* 475.

SUNDRY INSECTS

Puss caterpillar

Blister beetles

There is a variety of other insects which may cause injury to the human integument. The body fluid of certain kinds of beetles causes cutaneous blisters, and the caterpillars of certain moths (Fig. 20) and butterflies release toxins from body hairs, resulting in various degrees of urticaria. Generally, there is local burning and stinging in the affected area, and except for those insects which produce urticaria, the clinical problems are relatively small. There is usually no ulceration of the initial lesion, and systemic reactions are rare. Treatment involves topical application of palliative substances.

SELECTED REFERENCES

Lehmann, C. F., Pipkin, J. L., and Ressman, A. C. 1955. Blister beetle dermatosis. *A.M.A. Arch. Dermatol., 71:* 36.

Lucas, T. A. 1942. Poisoning by *Megalopype opercularis* ("puss caterpillar"). *J.A.M.A., 119:* 877.

McMillan, C. W., and Purcell, W. R. 1964. Hazards to health: the puss caterpillar, alias woolly slug. *New England J. Med., 271:* 147.

JELLYFISH

Portuguese man-of-war   *Physalia*

Clinical Picture. All jellyfish have stinging or nettle structures which release toxic substances when introduced into human skin. The effects of their sting depend on the nature and amount of toxin and the sensitivity of the patient. Although most jellyfish species produce stinging, burning sensations of the skin, the most dangerous effects are caused by the so-called Portuguese man-of-war, whose toxin may produce severe systemic reactions.

The toxin of this jellyfish has several fractions, the most serious of which seems to be a neurotoxin. When a patient is stung, there is intense pain that accompanies the stinging and burning sensations. Blood pressure may drop quickly, the pulse increases, and breathing may be labored. Urticaria, edema, chest pains, nausea, and muscle pains develop, the latter becoming spastic and may eventually become tetanic. Depending on the sensitivity of the patient, central nervous system depression may ensue, along with cardiac and respiratory failure.

Life Cycle. The patient ordinarily contacts the stinging tentacles of the jellyfish either accidentally while swimming or with disregard on

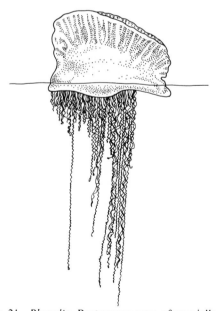

FIG. 21. *Physalia,* Portuguese man-of-war jellyfish.

the beach. The tentacles are extremely long, sometimes up to 100 feet, and even dead jellyfish on the beach have the capacity to sting if touched. Countless number of Portuguese men-of-war (Fig. 21) wash up on the South Atlantic and Gulf Coast beaches each year, usually in the fall.

Diagnosis. If a patient makes the contact on the beach, he is generally aware that he has had jellyfish sting. If the patient is stung when swimming a considerable distance from unseen jellyfish, he would be of no assistance in establishing diagnosis. In such a case stinging, burning sensations from the fiery, welt lesions (usually in linear fashion around the body or limbs) indicate jellyfish sting.

Treatment. Symptoms develop very quickly so that haste is of utmost importance. In addition to symptomatic measures, the best known treatment involves alcoholic baths; the action of the toxin is destroyed by alcohol.

Post-Treatment Advice. Patients should be urged to learn to recognize the bluish-colored Portuguese man-of-war and also to carry a supply of alcohol to the beach when these animals are plentiful at certain times of the year.

SELECTED REFERENCES

Frachtman, H. J., and McCollum, W. T. 1945. Portuguese Man-of-war stings. *Amer. J. Trop. Med., 25:* 499.

Ioannides, G., and Davis, J. H. 1965. Portuguese Man-of-war stinging. *Arch. Dermatol., 91:* 448.

STINGRAY

Clinical Picture. The effects in a patient stung by a ray are connected both with the wound or laceration and the venom introduced into the body. The rays have a rigid, serrated caudal spine (or stinger), surrounded by an integumentary sheath which contains the toxin. The wound—either a puncture or laceration (depending on what angle the fish strikes the patient)—is most often located on the feet or legs, less often on the trunk, and commonly on the hands and arms of commercial fishermen. The effects of the toxin vary, but in all cases are immediate and include exquisite pain, burning, throbbing and numbness of the stung area of the body. In some patients there is profuse sweating, muscle spasms, nausea, respiratory difficulties, and paralysis. Secondary infection may follow, and the wound is slow to heal.

Life Cycle. Stingray wounds are due to accidental intrusion on the privacy of the ray, which customarily lies buried in the muddy or sandy bottom off beaches or in inlets. The ray lifts up his tail and drives the spine into the patient.

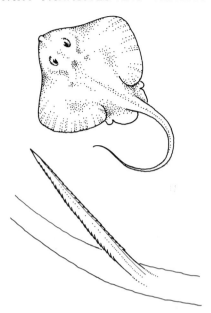

FIG. 22. Stingray; lower figure is enlargement of the ray's serrated spine.

Diagnosis. There is no problem in diagnosis when commercial fishermen are stung while emptying their nets or seines (the fisherman knows what has stung him!). The problem in diagnosis is when a patient has been stung and has not seen the ray. This occurs when wading or bathing or possibly at night when flounder fishing. If the stinger is still in the wound, recognition of the ray's spine (Fig. 22) establishes the diagnosis. If the patient has not seen what has stung him and if the spine is not in the wound, the nature of the puncture or laceration and the immediate clinical symptoms should suggest stingray contact.

Treatment. There is no antitoxin for stings due to rays. Treatment involves symptomatic measures and those directed against healing of the wound and preventing bacterial infection. Because the spine has recurved teeth, its removal from the patient may require incision and suturing. Antiseptic and antibiotic measures should be directed against the wound, and tetanus toxoid is advisable. In severe cases treatment for shock may be necessary. A variety of analgesics have been used to combat pain, but it is interesting to note that there have been a few cases where the injection of formalin directly into the wound resulted in dramatic, immediate cessation of pain and in rapid healing of the wound. In one unpublished case soaking the arm in vinegar for only a few minutes also brought dramatic relief, even though the sting was about an hour old.

Post-Treatment Advice. Patients should be advised about the risk involved when going into areas known to have stingrays.

SELECTED REFERENCE

Halstead, B. W., and Bunker, N. C. 1953. Stingray attacks and their treatment. *Amer. J. Trop. Med. & Hyg., 2:* 115.

SNAKEBITE

Rattlesnakes

Cottonmouths or water moccasins

Coral snakes

Copperheads

Clinical Picture. In all snakebites the wound is relatively unimportant compared to the effects of toxins which may be introduced into the integument of the patient. Although the nature of the toxins of poisonous snakes is generally imperfectly known, most are complex mixtures of a variety of substances, the most important of which are neurotoxic and hemotoxic materials. The clinical picture of snakebite depends on the character, amount and potency of toxin introduced, as well as the age of the patient.

Although neurotoxin produces considerable pain at the bite site, there is little or no swelling or discoloration around the bite. Neurotoxin is very fast-acting and produces such effects as nausea, headache, muscular weakness, prostration, and facial paralysis. Death may ensue because of respiratory failure due to toxic effect on the respiratory center in the brain.

When the chief component of snake venom is hemorrhagic, there is immediate pain, swelling, and discoloration at the bite site. These signs and symptoms intensify and extend to other parts of the body as the toxin is absorbed. Nausea, fatigue, and a feeling of suffocation develop in the patient. There is endothelial and small blood vessel damage by the toxin, resulting in considerable internal hemorrhage, and death is the result of circulatory collapse.

Although every poisonous snake has both neurotoxin and hemotoxin in its venom, usually one or the other predominates. Other substances, such as hyaluronidase, proteases, and coagulation and anticoagulation factors, have also been identified in the complex mixture.

Life Cycle. Snakebite is usually accidental to the patient but not to the snake. Snakes inhabit many kinds of ecologic situations, and every case of snakebite is potentially a medical emergency.

Diagnosis. The poisonous snakes in the United States are rattlesnakes, copperheads, cottonmouths or water moccasins, and coral snakes. The patient oftentimes has the opportunity to identify the snake or possibly has captured or killed it and brought the specimen in for identification. If none of the foregoing has been accomplished, then the bite marks and occurrence of early signs and symptoms are of considerable diagnostic importance in establishing whether a poisonous snake was involved and, secondly, whether neurotoxin or hemotoxin has been predominantly introduced into the patient. In the United States coral snakes have predominantly neurotoxin, whereas all other poisonous snakes have hemotoxin as the chief component of the venom.

If a poisonous snake has bitten the patient, an examination of the wound marks will show 1 or 2 puncture points of the fangs, as well as marks of the smaller teeth of the snake (Fig. 23A). The latter show as rows of dots or as scratches. If a poisonous snake had bitten with only one fang, then only a single, large puncture point is present. Moreover, some snakes, such as the coral, bite in such a fashion that there may be multiple fang marks. Although the bite pattern of a poisonous snake may at times be obscure, that of a nonpoisonous snake exhibits either rows of small punctures or rows of scratches but always without large fang puncture points (Fig. 23B).

If fang marks are present, this indicates that a poisonous snake has struck the patient, and the chief toxin introduced can be predicted,

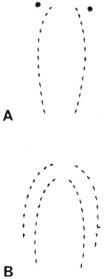

FIG. 23. Diagrammatic sketches of wound markings in snakebite: (A) poisonous snake marks showing fang puncture points; (B) non-poisonous snakebite marks. (After Werler's *Poisonous Snakes and First Aid Treatment of Their Bites*, Texas Game and Fish Commission, Austin, Texas.

even though the patient and/or the physician have not observed or identified the snake. The effects to the patient will vary (depending on many factors), but generally neurotoxin causes considerable pain but minimal swelling and discoloration, whereas hemotoxin produces pain, swelling and discoloration at the bite site. If several hours have passed since the patient was bitten, the signs and symptoms described above are quite characteristic.

Treatment. There is no unanimous agreement in the management of snakebite, and the handling of a case depends on many factors— among which are what first-aid measures were administered before seeing a physician and what the clinical status of the patient is when the doctor first confronts him. The most important factor is time, since the critical period following snakebite is the first 48 hours.

Of initial prime importance is determining the emotional status of the patient and reassuring him that treatment is effective. It is also important to establish the time the snake bit while the patient is still able to communicate. He should be transported by litter, and drinking of alcohol should be avoided, since both muscular activity and alcohol increase absorption of toxin. As most bites are on the arm and leg, these should be immobilized and a light tourniquet placed a few inches between the bite and the heart. The tourniquet should be loosened for a minute or two every 15 minutes. Ornaments or shoes should be removed immediately from the bitten limb.

A single, small incision over each fang mark, followed by suction (under sterility of the bite area and the commercial kit) is recommended by many, but only within the first 30 minutes after the bite. Under no circumstances should multiple incisions be made.

The physician should immediately render a judgment as to the potential severity of the case in relation to the time elapsed since the snakebite, noting the extent of edema and erythema around the bite and the systemic involvement. The most important therapeutic measure is the proper administration of antivenom at the earliest possible moment. Antihemotoxin is commercially available in the United States, and antineurotoxin is usually available from most large zoos. There are no strict rules regarding antivenom therapy, but rather this is based on the severity of the case and the clinical judgment of the physician. The important point is (following sensitivity testing and desensitization, if necessary) to administer an initial, large dose of antivenom (the smaller the body, the larger the dose). In severe cases with systemic symptoms, antivenom is given intravenously, otherwise by the subcutaneous or intramuscular route. Some authorities advocate a combination of routes.

Two other measures important in the management of snakebite are the injection of tetanus toxoid at the earliest possible moment and the administration of a broad-spectrum antibiotic.

Cryotherapy should be avoided, since this works against the passage of antivenom to the affected area and the dilution of the venom into the circulation.

Emergency measures, such as treatment for shock, blood transfusions, artificial respiration and tracheotomy, may be required in severe cases.

Post-Treatment Advice. Patients who (due to their occupation or recreation activities) run a high risk of snakebite should be advised to carry on their person a snakebite kit and should be instructed as to its use.

SELECTED REFERENCES

Lockhart, W. E. 1965. Treatment of snakebite. *J.A.M.A., 193:* 336.

Parrish, H. M. 1964. Texas snakebite statistics. *Texas State J. Med., 60:* 592.

——, Goldner, J. C., and Silberg, S. L. 1965. Snakebites in children and adults. *Pediatrics, 36:* 251.

Werler, J. E. 1963. Poisonous snakes of Texas and first aid treatment of their bites. *Bull. No. 31, Austin, Texas Fish and Game Commission.*

chapter three

INTESTINAL PARASITES

In addition to its various operational functions, the human intestinal tract is a conduit which provides loci for many parasitic organisms. These parasites include protozoans, trematodes, cestodes and nematodes. Most of them gain entrance into the gut by fecal contamination of food, water or fingers. Some intestinal parasites, however, first enter the body via skin penetration by the larval stage of the parasite and, after various migrational routes through tissue, mature in the intestine.

The effect of intestinal parasites on the human host varies from little or no damage to very severe consequences. In most cases parasitic burden determines symptomatology. Tissue erosion, ulceration, blockage, toxic effects, anemia and nutritional problems are among the many results of intestinal parasitism. Ectopic location of the parasites themselves (or the distribution of their larvae to extraintestinal sites) is the most damaging side of primary intestinal parasites.

Diagnosis is based on the morphologic recognition of the parasite itself or some stage in its life cycle. This can be accomplished by microscopic examination of fecal samples in most instances or—in the case of extraintestinal infection—of tissue.

AMEBIASIS

Entamoeba histolytica

Clinical Picture. Intestinal amebiasis denotes the presence in the large intestine of the protozoan *Entamoeba histolytica,* which is an actual or potential pathogen. The clinical picture in man is protean and varies according to the case—from the so-called carrier state (in which few or no symptoms occur) to such serious conditions as bloody, mucoid diarrhea, or dysentery. Active cases are generally considered as acute or chronic. Any bouts of diarrhea or dysentery accompanied by intestinal pain (especially in the lower right quadrant and in the absence of bacillary signs and symptoms) should suggest amebiasis. Chronic amebiasis is usually characterized by multiple bouts of diarrhea over some time. Constipation in between diarrhetic bouts is not uncommon. Such a patient complains of feeling dull, tired, and other nondescript feelings. Since the clinical picture of intestinal amebiasis is not sufficiently clear, the rule of thumb is to suspect all intestinal disturbances as being possibly amebic.

Life Cycle. A patient becomes infected by ingesting the resistant cyst stage of the parasite. This may be in or on contaminated food, drink, or fingers. In the patient the ameba may exist as either an active, vegetative and invasive form—the *trophozoite*—or as an encysted, nonactive, noninvasive *cyst* stage. There are intermediate morphologic stages between the trophozoite and cyst forms. The trophozoites are recovered from loose stools, whereas the cysts are characteristic of formed stools from carrier cases. The trophozoites may invade and colonize any portion of the large bowel, but this happens most frequently in the cecal area. The invasion of the mucosa results in small pinpoint lesions with raised edges. In further colonization the lesions may spread laterally in the mucosa and become so-called flask-shaped. On occasion, the lesions may penetrate the muscularis mucosa layer of the gut and then spread further in the submucosa. Confluence of lateral colonizations may result in necrosis and sloughing of the areas isolated from vascular supply.

In light or chronic cases where little or no tissue invasion takes place, the trophozoites become inactive, round up and secrete a cyst around themselves. The nuclei in such cysts then go on to divide, and in the case of *E. histolytica* the cysts are characteristically quadrinucleate when fully formed and typically found in formed stools of patients.

During active cases in which fecal material is moved quickly out of the gut, there is insufficient time for encystment to take place, so the trophozoite stage characterizes loose stools. However, the trophozoites do not play a part in the transmission of the infection from patient to patient, because they do not survive the outside environment. Even if they were ingested immediately, they would not survive passage through the upper intestinal tract. The patient passing cysts in his stool is therefore the important focal point as far as transmission is concerned.

Although there are no important reservoir hosts of this human pathogen, there are related amebae in many other kinds of animals. Out-breaks of active cases are usually due to contaminated water sources, whereas most other cases are connected with the fecal contamination of food with amebic cysts. Food handlers play an important part in the epidemiology of the infection.

Diagnosis. Demonstrating *E. histolytica* from a patient is among the most difficult tasks in diagnostic medical parasitology. One of the reasons for this is that there are at least five other species of amebae that may be present in the human gut, and *E. histolytica* must be distinguished from them. Moreover, diagnostic confusion often results when viewing such things as epithelial cells, macrophages, plant cells and artifacts in a stool sample. Because of these factors, it is a good idea for a beginning student to work up competence in recognizing *E. histolytica* alone before considering the many other things with which it can be confused. The latter will be dealt with at the end of this chapter.

The only valid diagnostic method is the direct microscopic examination of stools or proctoscopic samples of suspected colonic lesions. Although certain morphologic features are characteristic of *E. histolytica,* the general rule should be *not* to rely on any one feature, but rather to examine as many different organisms as possible before a definite conclusion is reached. The reason for this is that many features may be quite variable, rather than being as static as has been taught in the past. Moreover, the microscopic diagnosis of intestinal amebiasis is highly correlated with the training and competence of the person examining the sample, and this factor should be kept in the mind of the physician requesting an examination of a stool or proctoscopic sample.

Trophozoites are most likely recovered from diarrhetic stools and proctoscopic aspirates, whereas cysts are normally recovered from formed stools. Such samples are examined microscopically in saline preparations and by means of several supravital and permanent stains. The latter means of examination are the most rewarding.

The trophozoite of *E. histolytica* has a granular cytoplasm which may include ingested erythrocytes but lack bacteria in fresh specimens. The nucleus of the ameba usually has a small, centrally-located karyosome and a fine peripheral ring of chromatin in the nuclear membrane (Fig. 24A). In the spherical cyst stage the nuclear characteristics of *E. histolytica* remain the same as those in the trophozoite, but there are 1 to 4 nuclei in each cyst (Fig. 24B), depending on maturity. Also, depending on maturity, the cyst stage may exhibit rod-shaped chromatoidal bodies which characteristically have rounded ends.

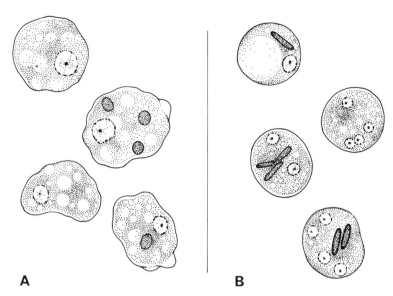

A   B

Fig. 24. *Entamoeba histolytica*: (A) trophozoites, two amebae having ingested erythrocytes; (B) cysts, three of which have chromatoidal bodies.

Intestinal amebiasis is cosmopolitan in geographic distribution, although the disease generally is of more severe nature in the tropics. It is emphasized that a single negative microscopic examination has no significance, and final negative diagnosis can be made only upon several examinations over some days. From the practical standpoint, the question of nonpathogenic *E. histolytica*-like parasites or nonpathogenic *E. histolytica* ought best to be ignored, and any *E. histolytica*-like organism should be considered potentially pathogenic and a patient with such be treated.

Treatment. There are many useful drugs in the management of intestinal amebiasis—among them various antibiotics, quinolines, arsenicals and bismuth compounds. To control diarrhea, antibiotics such as oxytetracycline or paromomycin are given, whereas diodohydroxyquin is administered either as an eliminative drug or in chronic cases. Since any patient having intestinal amebiasis runs the danger of developing amebic abscesses in deeper tissue (such as the liver and lungs), some feel it is important to give a patient drugs for possible undetected extraintestinal amebiasis. Since the above compounds are not sufficiently active in this respect, emetine has been used with this in mind—being active against both intestinal and extraintestinal amebiasis. It is, however, an extremely toxic compound which should be used with extreme caution. Chloroquine is a very useful drug for liver amebiasis, but its action against intestinal involvement is minimal.

Post-Treatment Advice. Any patient with intestinal amebiasis has had his food or drink contaminated with fecal material containing *E. histolytica* cysts. Patients from rural areas having no municipal water supply or sewage disposal system should be advised of the proper disposal of human excretory waste and a safe water source. Travelers to under developed countries who take their meals in public restaurants should be warned to avoid various uncooked foods (such as salads) which run a high risk of harboring amebic cysts.

SELECTED REFERENCES

Brooke, M. M., et al. 1964. Amebiasis: Laboratory Diagnosis. *Public Health Service Publication No. 1184, Introduction and Parts I, II and III.*

Faust, E. C. 1961. The multiple facets of *Entamoeba histolytica* infection. *Int. Rev. Trop. Med., 7:* 4.

Shaffer, J. G., Shales, W. H., and Radke, R. A. 1965. *Amebiasis: A Biomedical Problem.* 172 pp., Charles C. Thomas, Springfield, Illinois.

Wilmot, A. J. 1962. *Clinical Amoebiasis.* 166 pp., F. A. Davis Company, Philadelphia.

FASCIOLOPSIASIS

Giant intestinal fluke   *Fasciolopsis buski*

Clinical Picture. The effects of infection with this intestinal fluke depend on the number of worms in the gut. The adult worms attach to the mucosa of the duodenum and jejunum, resulting in inflammation, tissue erosion, and oftentimes hemorrhage and ulceration. As many as several thousand worms have been recovered from a single case, and such cases usually mimic peptic ulcer. In severe and chronic repetitive cases, general toxicity may result with edema of the face and abdomen. Eosinophilia up to 60 % is not unusual, and there may be general nutritional deficiencies, such as anemia. Some cases have been fatal.

Life Cycle. The infective cyst of this parasite is called the *metacercaria,* which is really an encysted, immature worm. This stage requires ingestion by a patient and happens inadvertently in several countries of the Far East when certain water plants (on which the fluke is encysted) are eaten. Upon entering the stomach, the cyst wall is dissolved, and after a month or two the young worms develop to maturity in the small intestine. The hermaphroditic flukes are thick, fleshy and large (7 mm)—as far as trematodes are concerned. In an infected case, the eggs of the worms are released in the gut and passed in the feces.

The eggs are relatively large and nonembryonated when voided from a patient. For further development, incubation of the eggs in water is

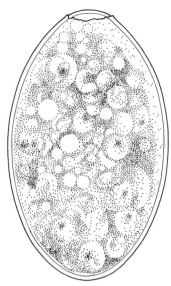

FIG. 25. *Fasciolopsis buski* egg

necessary. After a few weeks, a ciliated organism, the *miracidium,* develops in the egg and then hatches through the *operculum,* or lid. The free-living, motile miracidium must then penetrate a susceptible aquatic snail for additional development of the worm. Once inside the snail tissues, various larval multiplications occur, the end result being many active organisms—*cercariae*—which are periodically released in large numbers from the snail into the water. These cercariae then encyst on various aquatic plants, and when ingested by a patient, infection ensues. In addition to humans such animals as hogs and dogs are naturally infected with this worm.

Diagnosis. Since the clinical picture is not clear-cut (as is true with almost all helminthic infections), diagnosis is based on the microscopic identification of the worm egg in a stool specimen. This may be done directly from a stool sample or by using concentration methods. The egg is relatively large, ellipsoidal, nonembryonated, and has a small operculum, or lid, at the narrow end (Fig. 25). The adult worms are sometimes seen in stool specimens or in vomitus.

Treatment. Satisfactory treatment is accomplished by giving either hexylresorcinol or tetrachlorethylene on an empty stomach, followed by a saline purge a few hours later. Both of these drugs have also had wide usage in the treatment of certain intestinal nematode infections to be considered later.

Post-Treatment Advice. Persons who travel to known endemic areas should be cautioned in regard to the consumption of uncooked, aquatic plants.

SELECTED REFERENCES

Barlow, C. H. 1925. The life cycle of the human intestinal fluke *Fasciolopsis buski. Amer. J. Hyg. Monograph Ser. No. 4*, 98 pp.
Sadun, E. H., and Maiphoom, C. 1953. Studies on the epidemiology of the human intestinal fluke, *Fasciolopsis buski,* in Central Thailand. *Amer. J. Trop. Med. &Hyg., 2:* 1070.

HETEROPHYIASIS

Heterophyid flukes $\begin{cases} Heterophyes\ heterophyes \\ Metagonimus\ yokagawi \end{cases}$

Clinical Picture. These tiny flukes attach to, and may invade, the mucosa of the small intestine. Most cases exhibit the usual symptoms of gastrointestinal upset. There may be degrees of erosion, ulceration and necrosis of the gut, but much less so than in fasciolopsiasis. When the adult worms invade the mucosa, they may lay their eggs in the lymphatics and mesenteric vessels instead of the gut lumen. Because the worms are so small, they may gain entrance into these vascular vessels. In such ectopic cases, the worms and/or their eggs end up in such locations as the central nervous system and heart, resulting in nervous tissue damage and cardiac insufficiency.

Life Cycle. Human infection results following ingestion of raw or improperly cooked fish harboring viable metacercarial cysts. Excystment takes place in the human gut, and the young worms develop to maturity in a month or two. The hermaphroditic worms eventually lay small eggs which are passed in the feces of the patient. When voided in the feces, the eggs already have a fully developed miracidium inside.

The miracidium does not hatch, but rather the egg with the miracidium inside requires ingestion by a suitable aquatic snail before further development of the worm occurs. After larval multiplication inside the snail, the cercariae are released into the water. If these cercariae contact suitable fresh-water or brackish fish (especially mullet), then encystment occurs, and metacercariae locate under the scales and in the flesh of the fish.

There are at least two closely related heterophyid flukes of man, and both are nonspecific in relation to a vertebrate host, occurring naturally in a wide variety of animals, such as the cat, dog, many fish-eating mammals, and even birds. Human infection occurs mostly in the Far and Middle East and certain parts of Eurasia.

Diagnosis. Microscopic identification of the small, operculated eggs from a stool sample is the basis for diagnosis of the infection. The eggs are relatively very small, have small shoulders at the operculated end, and contain a fully-developed miracidium (Fig. 26). The eggs of

FIG. 26. Heterophyid egg

the two species may be distinguished from each other, but this need
not be done on a practical basis, since the treatment of both infections
is similar. Differential diagnosis is required, however, from the Chinese
liver fluke infection of man, the eggs of which are also found in fecal
samples. This is not an easy differentiation to make and will be taken
up in a later chapter.

Treatment. Tetrachlorethylene and hexylresorcinol are the drugs
of choice and are administered as described for fasciolopsiasis.

Post-Treatment Advice. The thorough cooking of fish from endemic
areas serves as a preventive measure.

SELECTED REFERENCES

Africa, C. M., Garcia, E. Y., and de Leon, W. 1935. Intestinal heterophyiasis with cardiac involvement. *Philippine J. Public Hlth., 2:* 1.

Khalil, M. 1933. The life history of the human intestinal parasite, *Heterophyes heterophyes* in Egypt. *Lancet, 2:* 537.

INTESTINAL SCHISTOSOMIASES

Intestinal bilharziasis　　　　*Schistosoma mansoni*

Oriental schistosomiasis　　　*Schistosoma japonicum*

Clinical Picture. The effects of this blood fluke infection vary according to many factors. The age of the patient, the number of previous
exposures, the worm burden and the. number of eggs deposited in
tissue, and ectopic locations of the worm eggs all have influence on
the nature of a clinical case. One general feature of schistosomiasis is
that the eggs are responsible chiefly for the disease rather than the
worms themselves. However, before the adult stage of the worms is
reached, there are various clinical signs and symptoms which may
occur.

The infection is acquired by skin penetration of the larval worms
(*cercariae*) and on multiple exposures various degrees of dermatitis
result, usually as an itchy, petechial rash. The dermatitis lasts for only
a few days.

When the juvenile worms are in the lungs, there may be a bronchial cough for a few days, fever, general allergic symptoms, and eosinophilia.

Eventually the mature worms are found in the mesenteric venules, and the females deposit eggs in the finer vessels. In an initial infection most of the schistosome eggs work themselves out into the lumen of the gut and are voided in the feces. However, with time passage and/ or multiple infections many worm eggs are trapped in the gut by tissue reactions. During this period there develops abdominal pain and commonly bloody, mucoid diarrhea. The gut tissue becomes sensitized to the eggs, the intestine becomes inflamed and eventually fibrotic. In severe cases there is small blood vessel damage, abscesses, and polyp formation of the gut.

Accompanying the above events, many eggs are laid in the blood stream and consequently swept back to such organs as the liver. The typical reaction around the eggs is of the pseudotubercle type. In severe or multiple cases, there is enlargement of both the liver and spleen, increased portal pressure, and lassitude of the patient. Terminal cases show extreme emaciation, ascites, and liver cirrhosis.

Other complications arise when eggs and/or worms locate ectopically in many other parts of the body, especially the central nervous system and lungs.

In light primary cases there are usually only minor effects, such as bloody stools and lassitude. Schistosome infection is more severe in children than in adults, and individuals appear to develop degrees of immunity to repeated infections. As is true with so many helminthic infections, nutrition plays a considerable role in the outcome of infection.

Life Cycle. A patient is infected by skin penetration of the larval form of the fluke in water. This stage (the *cercaria*) is an active organism, having a bifurcate tail, and can penetrate unbroken human skin. After penetration and gaining entrance into the lymphatics, the cercariae are carried to the right side of the heart, then to the lungs, the left heart, and eventually end up in portal blood—maturing into male and female worms in the portal radicles of the liver. This whole process takes 6 to 10 weeks.

The worms then migrate to the smaller venous extremities of the mesenteric system where they mate, (Fig. 27A) and the females then begin egg deposition. The eggs are either voided in the fecal mass, trapped in tissue, or swept back to the liver and other organs.

Eggs that are released in the stools contain an active, fully-developed

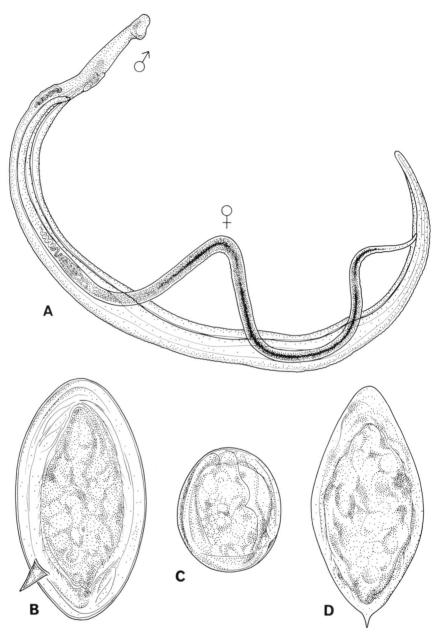

FIG. 27. Schistosomes: (A) adult male and female worms in copulation; eggs of (B) *Schistosoma mansoni,* (C) *Schistosoma japonicum,* (D) *Schistosoma haematobium.*

miracidium. This is a ciliated embryo that hatches when the eggshell ruptures upon entering water. The miracidium swims in water and must penetrate an appropriate snail host for further development of the fluke. When this is effected, a series of larval multiplications takes place within the snail, the end product being thousands of active cercariae released from the infected snail into the water.

There are two species of flukes causing intestinal schistosomiasis in man: *Schistosoma japonicum* of the Far East and *Schistosoma mansoni* of Africa, the Near East, South America and the West Indies. *S. japonicum* has a predilection for the superior mesenteric network, is found in many animals other than man, and is more serious than *S. mansoni* (since the female worms lay about 10 times more eggs). *S. mansoni* has a predilection for the inferior mesenteric veins (so that the large intestine and cecal area are more involved than the upper gut) and is not found to a significant degree in other animals.

Diagnosis. The microscopic identification of the characteristic schistosome eggs from the patient's feces is the basis for diagnosis. Both schistosome species have living miracidia inside the egg. *S. mansoni* eggs are ovoid and have a conspicuous lateral spine (Fig. 27B). *S. japonicum* eggs are subspherical and have an indistinct protuberance on one side (Fig. 27C). Neither species has an operculum, or lid. Since eggs may be difficult to recover in chronic cases, there are various concentration and hatching techniques that may be used to recover eggs. Also, in such cases many clinicians use rectal snips for diagnosis in which a piece of biopsied rectum is examined microscopically. Various immunologic tests have been devised for diagnosis, but it is too early to assess their real value; moreover, such tests are not routinely available.

Treatment. Despite the many years of search, there still is not available a highly useful chemotherapeutic agent against schistosomiasis. Antimony (in one form or another) has held the market since the first patient was ever treated for schistosomiasis. *S. japonicum* responds almost exclusively to potassium antimony tartrate. Stibophen and lucanthone hydrochloride are active against *S. mansoni* infections.

Post-Treatment Advice. The avoidance of contact with water in endemic areas should be stressed.

SELECTED REFERENCES

Kagan, I. G., and Pellegrino, J. 1961. A critical review of immunological methods for the diagnosis of bilharziasis. *Bull. Wld. Hlth. Org., 25:* 611.

Malek, E. A. 1961. The ecology of schistosomiasis. IN *Studies in Disease Ecology.* J. M. May, Ed. pp. 261–327, Hafner Publishing Company, Inc., New York.

Weller, T. H. 1947. The diagnosis of *Schistosoma mansoni* infections. *Amer. J. Trop. Med., 27:* 41.

World Health Organization. 1966. Chemotherapy of bilharziasis. *Wld. Hlth. Tech. Rep., No. 317,* pp. 3–71.

BEEF TAENIASIS

Beef tapeworm   *Taenia saginata*

Clinical Picture. The effect of beef tapeworm in the small intestine of a patient is nonspecific and—in fact—rather vague. General intestinal upset in the form of diarrhea, vomiting, vague "hunger pains," and weight loss may characterize the infection. There may be suggestions of liver damage, thought to be due to the absorption of toxic materials from the worm. As a result of chronic diarrhea of long duration, some patients may exhibit extreme nutritional and neurologic disturbances. In rare cases worms may ball up and obstruct the intestine, or portions of the worm may lodge in the appendix.

Life Cycle. A patient becomes infected by eating rare or raw beef containing viable larval cysts. These tapeworm larvae—called *cysticerci,* or *bladder worms*—may be located throughout the bovine but especially in skeletal muscle and the myocardium. Man and cattle are the only known hosts for the worm, and the infection occurs throughout the world. The transmission of this infection from man to cattle depends (as do so many other parasitic diseases) on defecation practices of the human.

The posterior segments of the worm (which may measure up to 30 feet) are filled with thousands of eggs. These ripe segments, or *proglittids,* detach from the main body of the worm and are usually voided intact and viable in the stool of the patient. On occasion some segments may migrate out of the anus irrespective of defecation and crawl on a patient's skin. There have been reported instances of proglottids from an armpit of a patient.

The fate of the proglottids is to disintegrate, liberating the eggs. When such eggs are ingested by grazing cattle, they hatch in the intestine and liberate viable embryos. These motile larvae (*oncospheres*) have six very pronounced hooks and penetrate the intestinal wall. They then gain entrance into lymph and blood and eventually filter out, mostly in skeletal muscle. Here they develop into cysticerci, which are fluid-filled sacs which bathe the head and the neck of the young tapeworm. To reach this infective stage in cattle, about two months are required after the bovine first ingests worm eggs.

Diagnosis. Beef tapeworm infection should be suspected in any patient with vague intestinal upset, especially if accompanied by abdominal pain, weakness and unexplained weight loss. Most cases exhibit practically no symptoms, and these patients usually turn themselves in because they note some white object in the stool or crawling on the skin. Diagnosis in the case of a patient who brings in a gravid

worm segment is a relatively simple matter. If the specimen is un-
preserved, it is pressed between two glass slides and held before a
strong light. The beef tapeworm has 15 to 20 (average 18) lateral
branches coming off the main stem of the uterus of the worm (Fig.
28A). If the specimen is preserved, it is stained and then examined for
the same characteristics.

Suspicion of beef tapeworm in other patients requires scotch tape
swabs of the perianal area. Although worm eggs erupted from dis-
integrated proglottids may be found in stool examinations, they do
not exist there in great density. The eggs are spherical and have a
thick shell with radial striations (Fig. 28B). Inside is the six-hooked
embryo, or oncosphere. The morphology of beef tapeworm eggs is
identical to that of pork tapeworm eggs and therefore is of no differential diagnostic value. Specific differential diagnosis is based on the
nature of the gravid proglottid and on the tapeworm head, or *scolex,*
which lacks hooks (Fig. 28C).

Treatment. Quinacrine has proved to be an effective and dependable
drug. Before its administration, however, proper patient preparation
is required. On the day before treatment, only liquids are allowed in
the patient's diet, followed by an evening purge or enema. In the
morning and on an empty stomach quinacrine is administered either
as a single oral dose or in divided doses over half an hour. Bicarbonate
may be necessary if the drug induces nausea in the patient. After about
two hours another purge is given, and the stool is examined for
worms.

Every effort should be made to find the head, or *scolex,* of the
tapeworm (not an easy or pleasant task, since it is about the size of a

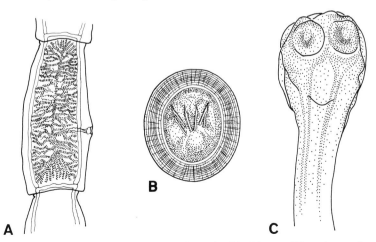

FIG. 28. *Taenia saginata*: (A) gravid proglottid; (B) egg; (C) scolex, or head

pinhead), as failure to expel the head results in the eventual development of a new entire worm.

If the head is not demonstrated (or it is good practice when it is,
since there may be more than one worm in the patient), weekly perianal examinations should be made for eggs for some months in order
to determine the success of treatment or the possible need for additional therapy.

Chlorsalicylamide and bithionol are proving to be useful drugs
against human taeniasis.

Post-Treatment Advice. Encouraging a patient not to eat rare steak
serves no purpose, the human dietary being what it is. Informing him
that the deep-freezing of beef for a day or two kills the bladder worms
may be more meaningful. Patients from farms should be advised of
the proper disposal of human excretory wastes.

SELECTED REFERENCES

Penfold, H. B. 1937. The signs and symptoms of *Taenia saginata* infestation. *Med. J.
Australia, 1:* 531.
Silverman, P. H., and Griffiths, R. B. 1955. A review of methods of sewage disposal in
Great Britain, with special reference to the epizootiology of *Cystercercus bovis. Ann.
Trop. Med. & Parasitol., 49:* 436.
Sodeman, W. A., and Jung, R. C. 1952. Treatment of taeniasis with quinacrine hydro-
chloride. *J.A.M.A., 148:* 285.

PORK TAENIASIS

Pork tapeworm   *Taenia solium*

Clinical Picture. Intestinal infection with the pork tapeworm usually
results in the same general symptomatology as beef tapeworm infection, except that intestinal disturbance may be more severe due to
more gut irritation by a crown of hooks on the head of the pork tapeworm.

Life Cycle. The life cycle and transmission factors of the pork tapeworm (except for one very important difference) are the same as the
beef tapeworm if one substitutes the pig for the cow as intermediate
host. The hog becomes infected by eating the worm eggs, and its bladder worms may be found in any part of the body, especially in such
areas as the tongue, shoulder muscles, and the heart. The important
difference is that, in addition to harboring adult worms, man may also
serve as intermediate host for the *cysticerci* or *bladder worms*. This
is the serious complication of pork tapeworm infection in man, and
it apparently also occurs in patients with no history of having had
adult worms. This aspect will be considered in the chapter on tissue

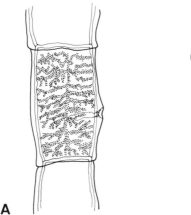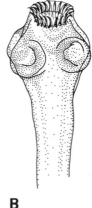

A   **B**

FIG. 29. *Taenia solium*: (A) gravid proglottid; (B) scolex, or head. (Egg of *T. solium* is identical to that of *T. saginata* (Fig. 28B).

parasites. Pork taeniasis is distributed especially in countries where pork is consumed insufficiently cooked or raw.

Diagnosis. The suspicion and diagnosis of pork tapeworm is similar to that of beef tapeworm, although it is surprising that larval infections of man are much more frequently reported than intestinal infection with the adult worm. It is important to note that a patient requiring surgical removal of bladder worms from his tissues should be examined and treated, if necessary, for adult worms in his intestine.

The eggs of pork tapeworm and beef tapeworm are identical and therefore of no specific differential value. However, the gravid proglottid of a pork tapeworm specimen (Fig. 29A) has less lateral uterine branches off the main stem (7 to 13, average 9), and diagnosis based on this structure is specific. An additional criterion is the fact that the pork tapeworm has a crown of hooks around the four powerful suckers of the head end of the worm (Fig. 29B), whereas the head of the beef tapeworm is unarmed.

Treatment. Quinacrine is effective against the adult worm and is administered in the same manner as described for beef tapeworm cases.

Post-Treatment Advice. Comments to an infected and treated patient are of a similar nature as expressed for beef tapeworm infection. In a patient harboring adult worms, the potential of autoinfection should be recognized, and the patient's cooperation for successful treatment should be strongly solicited.

SELECTED REFERENCES

Schwartzwelder, J. C. 1939. Clinical *Taenia* infection: an analysis of sixty cases. *J. Trop. Med. & Hyg.*, 42: 226.

Yoshina, K. 1934. On the subjective symptoms caused by the parasitism of *Taenia solium* and its development in man. *Taiwan Igakkai Zasshi, 33:* 14.

HYMENOLEPIASIS

Dwarf tapeworm   *Hymenolepis nana*

Clinical Picture. The dwarf tapeworm is a tiny cestode of the small intestine of man and rodents. The symptomatology depends on the number of worms in the gut and the age of the patient. General intestinal upset, including vague abdominal pain, irritability and mild diarrhea, may be part of the clinical picture. In children with a heavy worm burden, symptoms are of a more severe nature and include insomnia and epileptoid convulsions.

Life Cycle. Dwarf tapeworm infection is apparently mostly a man-to-man infection. The gravid proglottids of this worm rupture in the intestine, liberating their eggs, which are immediately infective when swallowed. No intermediate host is required, and the infection of another person (or the reinfection of a patient to himself) requires only the ingestion of the worm eggs. The swallowed eggs hatch in the small intestine, and the larva, or onchosphere, penetrates the intestinal villi, where it develops into a modified bladder worm, or *cysticercoid*. The larva is not fluid-filled (as is that of the beef and pork tapeworm larva), but rather has a solid tail-like structure connected to the inverted head and neck of the worm. The cysticercoid undergoes development for a few days and then breaks out into the lumen of the gut. Here it develops into a mature, adult tapeworm in a few weeks.

There is evidence that an untreated patient may be a constant source of infection to himself in one or two ways. Eggs may actually hatch in the intestine (rather than being voided in the feces), and this is followed by gut penetration of the oncosphere and the ensuing cycle. A patient may also reinfect himself by ingesting eggs by hand-to-mouth transmission or via fomites. Either type of autoinfection results in large worm loads in a patient. Dwarf tapeworm has a cosmopolitan geographic distribution.

Diagnosis. A stool examination provides diagnosis, either by direct microscopic examination of a fecal sample or by stool concentration methods. The egg of the dwarf tapeworm is characteristic, being spherical or subspherical in shape and with a very thin shell (Fig. 30). The six-hooked embryo, or oncosphere, within the egg has two polar thickenings from which arise filamentous strands.

The proglottids of the dwarf tapeworm are also diagnostic but are

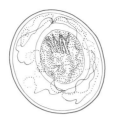

FIG. 30. *Hymenolepsis nana* egg

rarely found in the stools of untreated patients and are therefore of little diagnostic value.

Treatment. Quinacrine is used in the same manner as outlined for beef and pork tapeworm infections. Since dwarf tapeworm eggs are immediately infective, proper precaution should be expressed in terms of personnel involved with the patient and his stools.

Post-Treatment Advice. Hygienic habits, the proper disposal of excrement, and the importance of autoinfection should be stressed.

SELECTED REFERENCES

Chandler, A. C. 1922. The species of *Hymenolepsis* as human parasites. *J.A.M.A., 78:* 636.

Sunkes, E. J., and Sellers, T. F. 1937. Tapeworm infestation in the southern United States. *Amer. J. Public Hlth., 27:* 893.

DIPHYLLOBOTHRIASIS

Broad fish tapeworm   *Diphyllobothrium latum*

Clinical Picture. As is true with all tapeworm infections of the human intestinal tract, those with the broad fish tapeworm may involve general intestinal upset, vague abdominal pain, diarrhea, nausea, and weight loss. This worm may measure up to 30 feet long, and it is truly amazing that so many patients play host to such a large creature with relatively little discomfort. On the other hand, there is a serious side to infection with this tapeworm, and this involves the actual or potential development of anemia. This condition seems more prevalent in certain Nordic groups and apparently results from the worm competing for vitamin B_{12} from the human gut.

Life Cycle. A patient becomes infected by eating raw or improperly cooked fish, usually of the pike, pickerel or walleye variety. The life cycle of the broad fish tapeworm is complex compared to those of other cestodes which infect man. In addition to humans many animals whose diet includes the consumption of raw, fresh-water fish may be naturally infected with the adult tapeworm. These include

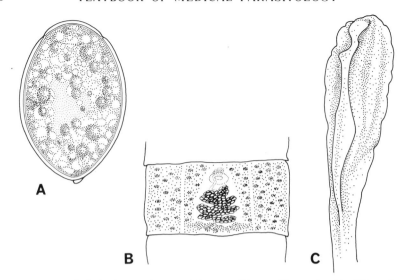

FIG. 31. *Diphyllobothrium latum*: (A) egg; (B) gravid proglottid; (C) scolex, or head.

bears, mink, seals, dogs and cats. The geographic distribution of the infection is widespread, but human infection is prevalent in those areas where fresh-water fish constitute an important item in the diet of the human population.

The mature segments, or proglottids, of the broad fish tapeworm are unlike those of other tapeworms of man in that the eggs of the worm are continuously released through the uterine pore. As many as a million eggs are voided in the feces of a patient per day. An additional difference of the broad fish tapeworm is that the egg is very trematode- or fluke-like, having an operculum, or lid, at one end. Uncleaved eggs in feces require incubation in fresh water environments for a week or two, after which a ciliated larva—the *coracidium* —hatches through the opened lid.

The coracidium swims and spins around in the water in much the same manner as a protozoan organism and requires ingestion by certain copepod crustaceans for further development to take place. Within the body cavity of the copepod the oncosphere develops into an elongate, sacculate type of larva called the *procercoid*.

The procercoid stage requires ingestion by various types of fish for continuation of this tapeworm cycle. These may be small fry of the pike or pickerel type or other kinds of fish which are themselves eaten by larger fish. In any event the final result is that the procercoid is eventually liberated in the gut of an adult fish and migrates to its muscles. Here it elongates and develops into a *plerocercoid* or *sparganum* larva. When viable spargana are present in improperly cooked fish, they develop into adult tapeworms in the human intestinal tract after a couple of months.

Diagnosis. Since the eggs are usually plentiful in an infected patient, direct microscopic examination of a fecal sample is usually sufficient for diagnosis. The egg is ovoid, nonembryonated, has a pronounced lid, or operculum, at one end, and a knob-like structure at the end opposite the lid (Fig. 31A). Other features of diagnostic importance include the rosette appearance of the uterus in a gravid proglottid (Fig. 31B), and the presence of two sucking grooves, or bothria, on the scolex (Fig. 31C).

Treatment. Quinacrine is the drug of choice, and its administration and patient preparation is similar to that described for beef tapeworm infection.

Post-Treatment Advice. To advise a patient to eat properly cooked fish would be of no practical value if he likes it the other way. With respect to the freezing of fish, it should be pointed out that plerocercoid larvae may survive low temperatures for long periods of time and that packaged, frozen fish may be a source of infection.

SELECTED REFERENCES

von Bonsdorff, B. 1956. *Diphyllobothrium latum* as a cause of pernicious anemia. *Exp. Parasitol., 5:* 207.
Weinstein, P. P., and Appleget, J. G. 1952. Some observations on *Diphyllobothrium latum* from Shagwa Lake, Minnesota. *Amer. J. Trop. Med. & Hyg., 1:* 302.

ASCARIASIS

Giant intestinal roundworm *Ascaris lumbricoides*

Clinical Picture. As in most worm infections, the clinical picture of ascariasis depends on how many parasites are in the body and the location of the worms. A case of ascariasis involves both a tissue and intestinal phase of the worms. After initial infection the larval worms migrate to various tissues, but their presence is indicated mostly in the liver and lungs, particularly the latter. An infected patient may experience labored respiration, cough, fever, and transient eosinophilia. The larvae cause hemorrhagic areas which are infiltrated by various blood elements, particularly eosinophils. The pneumonitis syndrome later disappears as the larvae move into and mature into adult worms in the small intestine.

Although the adult nematodes in the intestine may reach a foot or so in length, symptoms related to this phase of the infection depend on how many worms are present and also how they behave in that location. With a light infection the patient exhibits gastrointestinal upset, colic, and nervous symptoms. In more serious circumstances the worms may ball up in the intestinal tract, resulting in blockage symptoms.

Equally serious is the propensity for the adult worm to migrate from its usual location in the small intestine. Such migrations may be down and out the anus or up and through the mouth and/or nose. In other cases worms may migrate to and occlude the bile duct (resulting in jaundice of the patient) or even pierce the intestinal wall and initiate peritonitis. Occlusion of the appendix is also not rare.

Life Cycle. A patient becomes infected by ingesting worm eggs containing infective larvae inside. The eggs hatch in the small intestine, the larvae are liberated and then penetrate the intestinal wall and gain entrance into the vascular system. They then enter the liver, heart, and finally the lungs. It is in the latter organ that they reside for a week or so and induce pneumonitis reactions. Following this, they ascend the respiratory tree to the pharynx, where the larvae are swallowed and then mature into adult worms in the small intestine after several weeks.

Eggs are released in the feces in a nonembryonated condition and require incubation in the soil for a few weeks in order that the infective larva may develop. In children ascariasis seems to be more of a hand-to-mouth kind of transmission, whereas in adults the contamination of food with infective eggs is probably the chief source of infection. The eggs are highly resistant and can remain viable for months and years under the proper physical-chemical conditions. Ascariasis is widely distributed in human populations and especially prevalent in tropical areas.

Diagnosis. The pneumonitis phase of ascariasis cannot be diagnosed with certainty. Successive radiographs of lungs often show a shifting, mottling effect, and this feature—coupled with the clinical picture as described (especially eosinophilia)—should certainly suggest ascariasis. Such a person should be examined several weeks later when the worms are mature in his gut and passing eggs which can be detected in the stools.

Mature infections can be diagnosed without difficulty by the microscopic identification of the egg in a stool sample, although a distinction must be made between fertile and infertile eggs.

The fertile egg (Fig. 32A) is ovoid, nonembryonated, and the eggshell has an outside rugose layer of material. The infertile egg (Fig. 32C) is ellipsoid, being longer and narrower than fertile eggs, and usually has a thinner outside coating. Both fertile and infertile eggs may be present in a stool sample without the outside mammillated layer (Figs. 32B & 32D). Eggs will obviously not be present if the infection is only with male worms, and in such cases radiographic detection is in order.

Treatment. There is no effective treatment against the larval phase of the infection, but this cannot usually be diagnosed anyway. Piperazine is the drug of choice for adult worms. Fasting before treatment and purgation after treatment (practiced in some other worm infections) is not necessary. The worms are passed in a living state and can be easily detected in the post-treatment stool. Treated patients

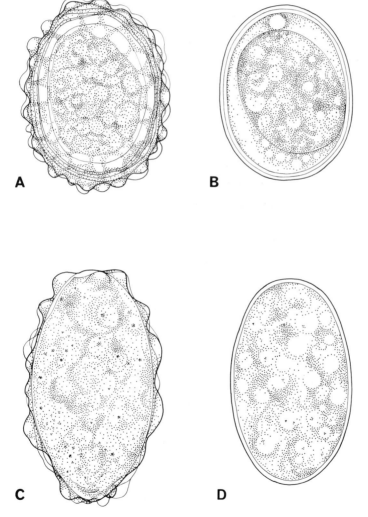

FIG. 32. *Ascaris lumbricoides* eggs: (A) fertile; (B) fertile egg without outside coat; (C) infertile; (D) infertile egg without mamillated outside layer.

should be advised to return several weeks later to be checked by stool examination for additional worms. These would result from the development and maturation of any larvae in tissues at the time of initial treatment.

Post-Treatment Advice. As with most parasites, ascariasis results from the improper disposal of human excretory wasts, and patients should be advised accordingly. This infection also rates high in the kind that is contracted by travelers to underdeveloped areas who do not avoid uncooked foods, such as salads.

SELECTED REFERENCES

Brown, H. W., and Stermann, M. M. 1954. Treatment of ascariasis with piperazine. *J. Pediatr., 45:* 419.

Jelliffe, D. B., and Jung, R. C. 1957. Ascariasis in children. *W. Indian Med. J., 6:* 113.

Ochsner, A., DeBakey, E., and Dixon, L. 1949. Complications of ascariasis requiring surgical treatment. *Amer. J. Dis. Child., 77:* 389.

Swartzwelder, J. C. 1946. Clinical ascariasis—an analysis of 202 cases in New Orleans. *Amer. J. Dis. Child., 72:* 172.

HOOKWORM INFECTION

Old World hookworm   *Ancylostoma duodenale*
American hookworm   *Necator americanus*

Clinical Picture. The nature of hookworm infection varies according to the worm load and the nutritional status of the patient. As in ascariasis, there is both a pneumonitis and intestinal phase of the infection. But unlike ascariasis there are also cutaneous aspects, since a patient becomes infected by skin penetration by the hookworm larvae living in the soil.

A dermatitis with burning and itching is usual, and with repeated exposures to larvae, hypersensitive reactions ensue, and the dermatitis may be intensified. Pneumonitis develops (as in ascariasis), but it is less severe and there is less propensity for hypersensitive reactions during this phase of the infection.

The adult nematodes in the small intestine actively attach to the epithelial lining of the gut, erode tissue, and suck blood. The effects of hookworms in the gut may vary from little or no symptomatology to severe anemia. A light worm burden may cause general gastrointestinal upset, diarrhea, colic and fever, whereas heavy worm loads or infections of long duration interfere with the nutrition of the patient and may drop the hemoglobin to critical levels.

Life Cycle. A patient becomes infected by the contact of his skin to infective larvae. After skin penetration, the larvae are eventually carried to the heart, enter the arterial circulation, and within a day or two filter out in the lung capillaries. After growth and development in the lungs for about a week, the larvae break into the alveolar sacs, ascend the respiratory tree, and are swallowed and then develop into mature hookworms in the small intestine in a month or two. Here the worms mate, and the female lays eggs which pass out in the feces of the patient. Under suitable conditions of the soil, the eggs develop and hatch into *rhabditiform* larvae, which then grow and develop further into the infective *filariform* larva of the worm. There are no reservoir hosts of human hookworm infection.

Diagnosis. The pneumonitis phase cannot be diagnosed with certainty, but if there is a history of dermatitis in a patient's body areas likely to have been in contact with soil, hookworm infection would be suspect, and the patient's stool ought to be examined several weeks later.

A stool examination is all that is required for mature hookworm infection, and the microscopic identification of the characteristic egg in the feces determines definite diagnosis. Human hookworm infection is a world-wide affair, but more prevalent in tropical and subtropical areas. There are two species which infect man as adult worms, but since their eggs are identical and their treatment similar, the distinction need not be made on a practical basis.

Human hookworm eggs are ovoid with bluntly rounded ends. The eggshell is extremely thin and transparent (Fig. 33). Eggs recovered from a stool sample usually exhibit embryologic cleavage to the 2 or 8-cell stage, but some eggs may be in morula form.

Treatment. There are several effective drugs against adult hookworms, but the one of choice seems to be tetrachlorethylene. If a coinfection of ascariasis exists, however, this drug should not be

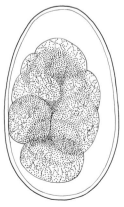

FIG. 33. *Ancylostoma duodenale* or *Necator americanus* egg

used initially, since it stimulates the *Ascaris* worms to migrate from their usual locations in the small intestine. In such cases the ascariasis should be treated first with piperazine and, after a cure, the patient can be treated for the hookworm by use of tetrachlorethylene.

Bephenium may be used in cases of double infection with hookworm and *Ascaris,* or with *Ancylostoma* alone, since it is more active against the latter than tetrachlorethylene. As with ascariasis, stools of patients treated for hookworm should be examined some weeks later for eggs resulting from the maturation of tissue larvae possibly present at initial therapy. Secondary treatment may be necessary, as well as general supportive therapy in the form of iron, high protein and high minerals.

Post-Treatment Advice. The proper disposal of human excrements should be stressed, particularly in areas which do not have a municipal sewage system and in patients whose occupation or habits require close contact with soil.

SELECTED REFERENCES

Scott, J. A. 1945. Hookworm disease in Texas. *Texas Rep. Biol. & Med., 3:* 558.
Stoll, N. R. 1962. On endemic hookworm, where do we stand today? *Exp. Parasitol., 12:* 241.
Weil, A. J. 1953. Hookworm infection as a diagnostic problem in New York City. *N.Y. State J. Med., 53:* 1085.

STRONGYLOIDIASIS

Threadworm   *Strongyloides stercoralis*

Clinical Picture. Although the acquisition of infection and life cycle within the body of a strongyloidiasis case and a hookworm case are similar, there are notable differences in the clinical picture of these nematode infections. When infective larvae penetrate human skin, there is itching and dermatitis but not to the degree found in hookworm cases. This is because the larvae linger for shorter periods of time in the cutaneous areas. Consequently, dermatitis in strongyloidiasis is usually very transient, unless there is secondary bacterial infection.

The larvae make the same heart-lung respiratory circuit as hookworm larvae so that a pneumonitis phase of strongyloidiasis also occurs. Once the adult worms mature in the small intestine, they locate deeply in the intestinal mucosa and cause protean gastrointestinal symptoms. Eosinophilia is characteristic, and a chief complaint seems to be epigastric pain. Allergic reactions, such as urticaria, are not unusual.

Life Cycle. A patient becomes infected by contact of his skin with soil containing the infective larvae. The migration of the larvae and their development to maturity in the body is similar to hookworm infection. Whereas hookworms attach to the intestinal epithelium of the gut and suck blood, in a strongyloidiasis case the nematodes are embedded in the mucosa and move around considerably in this tissue. The females lay eggs in the mucosa, and in very short order these hatch and develop into a type of larvae called rhabditiform. It is this larva that is characteristically passed in the stool of an infected patient.

One of the serious features of strongyloidiasis cases has to do with certain potential aspects of the life cycle within the body. This is connected with the problem of a patient's increasing his worm burden in the absence of additional infection from the outside environment. Such self-infection is called *autoinfection* and may occur in either of two ways. The rhabditiform larva (which is not infective to man), instead of being passed to the outside in the stool, may develop in the intestine into another type of larva called the filariform. This form of the nematode is infective, and within the gut it may penetrate tissue, take the lung-respiratory route, and develop to maturity in the small intestine. This course of events is referred to as *internal autoinfection.*

Another self-infection procedure is for the filariform larva to develop in fecal residue around the perianal region of the patient and then penetrate through the skin of this area. The migration route and development into new worms is similar to that described above.

When rhabditiform larvae are passed in the stool, their development into the infective filariform larva in the soil is similar to that of the hookworm cycle. There is a possible difference in the life cycles of hookworm and a *Strongyloides* worm at this point, however, in that the rhabditiform larva of the latter may develop into mature male and female worms in the soil. This free-living aspect of the cycle may go on for some time, and at certain points the rhabditiform larvae (instead of developing into adult free-living worms) transform into infective filariform larvae, which may then initiate infection when coming into contact with human skin.

Diagnosis. As is true with other nematodes of this type, the pneumonitis phase cannot be diagnosed with certainty. Gastrointestinal symptoms, coupled with epigastric pain and eosinophilia, should always suggest strongyloidiasis.

The microscopic identification of rhabditiform larvae (Fig. 34) in a stool sample is diagnostic. It is possible to distinguish this larva from

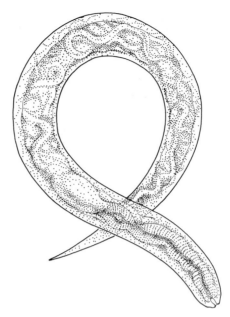

FIG. 34. *Strongyloides stercoralis* rhabditiform larva

the hookworm larva (which may on occasion develop precociously in the gut) by the former having a shorter buccal cavity. Some workers prefer duodenal aspirates over stool examinations for demonstration of the larva. Strongyloidiasis is cosmopolitan in geographic distribution, and there are no proven natural reservoir hosts for the infection.

Treatment. The chemotherapy of strongyloidiasis is not without difficulties. The most effective drug seems to be dithiazanine, but this compound is coming into disfavor. This is because some patients absorb the drug, resulting in severe reactions and sometimes fatalities. Another drug that may be used is pyrvinium pamoate. Some reports indicate that thiabendazole shows promise as a highly active drug for this infection, although it has not been licensed for human use as yet.

Post-Treatment Advice. The factors involved in the acquisition of hookworm infection should be pointed out with respect to strongyloidiasis. The importance of complete cure should be emphasized, particularly because of potential autoinfection.

SELECTED REFERENCES

Brown, H. W., and Perna, V. P. 1958. An overwhelming *Strongyloides* infection. *J.A. M.A., 168:* 1648.

Franz, K. H. 1963. Clinical trials with thiabendazole against human strongyloidiasis. *Amer. J. Trop. Med. & Hyg., 12:* 211.

Huchton, P., and Horn, R. 1959. Strongyloidiasis. *J. Pediatr., 55:* 602.

Yoeli, M., Most, H., Berman, H. H., and Scheinesson, G. P. 1963. The clinical picture and pathology of massive *Strongyloides* infection in a child. *Trans. Roy. Soc. Trop. Med. & Hyg., 57:* 346.

ENTEROBIASIS

Pinworm   *Enterobius vermicularis*

Clinical Picture. A variety of signs and symptoms have been ascribed to pinworm infection, but the only near-constant picture seems to be perianal itching and restlessness (particularly at night). The adult nematodes attach only superficially to the epithelium of the cecal area, and they do not suck blood as do hookworms. Consequently, gastrointestinal upset and tissue damage is minimal. It is not unusual, however, for worms to migrate into the vaginal area of females and initiate varying degrees of vaginitis.

Life Cycle. A patient acquires pinworm infection by ingesting the worm eggs containing infective larvae. This may be in a variety of ways, such as hand-to-mouth transmission, inhalation of eggs (followed by swallowing), and the handling of contaminated fomites or food. The infective larvae hatch out of the eggs in the small intestine and then migrate to the cecal area of the large bowel, where they mature and mate. This entire period from ingestion of eggs to maturation of worms takes 3 to 4 weeks.

The female nematodes do not usually release eggs in the gut but rather travel to the perianal region (particularly at night) and release their eggs there, usually by rupture of the worm body. The eggs are infective within a matter of hours after leaving the female worms.

Most patients become infected by close contact (in one form or another) with an infected case. If one member of a family is infected, it is quite a safe guess to anticipate the entire family will also come down with pinworm. This infection is cosmopolitan in geographic distribution, and there are no vertebrate hosts other than man.

There is no acquired immunity to pinworm infection, so an infected patient can continue to reinfect himself, either in a hand-to-mouth style, or simply by ingesting by some other means the eggs he is continuously passing. There is also some evidence that some eggs may hatch in the perianal region, and these larvae then re-enter the large intestine and mature into adult worms. This mode is called *retroinfection.*

Diagnosis. Because of the nature of the life cycle of the worm within the body, pinworm eggs are unlikely to be found in a regular stool examination. Consequently, the best means of diagnosis is by various modifications of the so-called scotch-tape method. This involves the pressing of cellophane tape on the perianal region, preferably early in the morning before a bath or bowel movement. The tape is then affixed to a slide and examined microscopically.

Several perianal swabs over successive days are highly rewarding compared to a single examination. Microscopic identification of the pinworm egg is diagnostic. It is ovoid but asymmetrically flattened on one side (Fig. 35). Most eggs have active larvae which are looped on themselves.

Treatment. Two highly effective drugs for pinworm infection are piperazine for 5 days or pyrvinium pamoate in split doses 5 days apart. There is little point in treating one individual of a family without determining possible infections in the other members. If this is not convenient, then the next best thing is to treat all members of the family, irrespective of their having been examined for pinworm.

Post-Treatment Advice. The importance of determining infections in the entire family (and possible entire family treatment) should be explained in terms of the life cycle of the worm.

It should also be emphasized to the patient that a complete "swab the deck" undertaking should be accomplished before and during treatment. A parent should also be advised of the high risk of pinworm infection that accompanies the current "slumber parties" of young children.

SELECTED REFERENCES

Beaver, P. C. 1949. Methods of pinworm diagnosis. *Amer. J. Trop. Med., 29:* 577.
Pryor, H. B. 1955. *Oxyuris vermicularis.* The most prevalent parasite encountered in the practice of pediatrics. *J. Pediatr., 46:* 262.
Swartzwelder, J. C. 1957. The effective use of piperazine for the treatment of human helminthiases. *Gastroenterology, 33:* 87.

TRICHURIASIS

Whipworm   *Trichuris trichiura*

Clinical Picture. The clinical status of a patient having whipworm infection varies according to the number of worms present in the large intestine. A few nematode worms result in little, if any, signs and symptoms. With moderate worm burdens there are various gastrointestinal disturbances, among which epigastric or abdominal pain seems more consistent than others. In severe cases there may be bloody stools, considerable erosion of the gut, anemia and rectal prolapse.

Life Cycle. A patient becomes infected by ingesting whipworm eggs

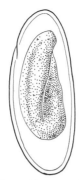

FIG. 35. *Enterobius vermicularis* egg

containing the infective larva. This is accomplished mostly by food contamination or by hand-to-mouth transmission from the soil.

After being swallowed, the eggs hatch in the small intestine. The liberated larvae develop further here (about a week) and then slowly migrate to the cecal area of the large bowel, where they mature into adult male and female nematode worms. In this area the thin anterior ends of the worms penetrate and remain attached to the mucosal lining of the gut. The entire cycle in the human body to this point takes about three months.

Eggs which are released from the female worms are voided in the fecal mass. Since they are released in an uncleaved condition, they require further development in the soil before an infective larva develops within the egg. This requires a few weeks under suitable environmental conditions.

The worms are long-lived in the human body, and indications are that they may release eggs up to several years. Man is the only host to this species, and although the infection is cosmopolitan in geographic distribution, it is more prevalent in warm, moist climates.

Diagnosis. The microscopic identification of the characteristic whipworm egg from a stool sample is all that is required for diagnosis. The egg is barrel- or lemon-shaped, nonembryonated, and has a bipolar appearance due to a transparent plug at each end (Fig. 36). Concentration methods of stool samples may be required to detect eggs in infections.

Treatment. Dithiazanine is highly effective against whipworm infection, but because of the drug's potential toxicity its use should be carefully deliberated. Pyrvinium pamoate is also effective and of less relative toxicity. In high-risk patients the use of high-retention enemas of hexylresorcinol results in clinical improvement of a case. As is true for strongyloidiasis, the management of whipworm infection awaits more useful chemotherapeutic agents.

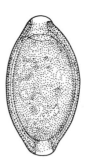

FIG. 36. *Trichuris trichiura* egg

Post-Treatment Advice. Since whipworm is an orally-acquired infection, the importance of adequate sewage disposal, the risk in eating uncooked foods in endemic areas, and personal hygiene should be emphasized.

SELECTED REFERENCES

Jung, R. C., and Beaver, P. C. 1952. Clinical observations on *Trichocephalus trichiuris* (whipworm) infestation in children. *Pediatrics, 8:* 548.
Swartzwelder, J. C. 1939. Clinical *Trichocephalus trichiuris* infection. *Amer. J. Trop. Med., 19:* 437.

SUNDRY INTESTINAL INFECTIONS

	Giardia lamblia
	Dientamoeba fragilis
	Entamoeba coli
	Endolimax nana
	Iodamoeba bütschlii
	Isospora
	Balantidium coli
Double-barreled tapeworm	*Dipylidium caninum*
Rat tapeworm	*Hymenolepis diminuta*

The following organisms (because they do not often occur in man, or because their pathogenesis is slight or questionable) are less important in the total picture of human parasites.

Giardiasis. *Giardia lamblia* is a small, flagellated protozoan of the human small intestine and is associated with variable effects. Some patients exhibit few (if any) symptoms that can definitely be related to its presence, whereas other patients show serious clinical conditions, such as voluminous mucoid diarrhea, epigastric pain, constipation, intestinal malabsorption, and urticaria.

A patient acquires the infection by ingesting the cyst stage of the organism, either in food or water or via the hand-to-mouth route. The cysts excyst in the duodenal region of the gut and undergo multiplication there. The trophozoite or vegatative stage is usually located in the intestinal crypts but may also occur and multiply in the biliary passages. The trophozoites are believed to attach to the intestinal epithelium by means of the adhesive discs of the organisms. Cysts of the organisms are released in formed stools of an infected patient.

Diagnosis is based on the morphology and characteristic movement of trophozoites from diarrhetic stools or on the cyst stage from stained stool samples.

The trophozoite (Fig. 37A) is pear-shaped, having an extremely thin body, the ventral side of which has two large, concave, adhesive discs. There are two prominent nuclei per trophozoite, and each trophozoite has deeply-staining, rod-like structures, as well as eight flagellae.

The cyst stage (Fig. 37B) is ovoid, and in stained specimens the contents have shrunk away from the thin cyst wall. Two or four prominent nuclei are present as well as the characteristic, rod-shaped structures. Giardiasis occurs far more often in children than in older age groups.

Quinacrine is a safe and effective drug, and the decision as to whether or not to treat should be based on what else seems to be wrong in the patient. In view of the pathogenic potential of this or-

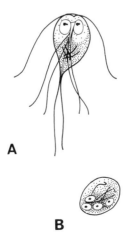

A

B

FIG. 37. *Giardia lamblia*: (A) trophozoite; (B) cyst

ganism it makes sense to treat unless other factors contraindicate the administration of the drug.

As with amebiasis, patients with giardiasis indicate that fecal contamination of food or water has taken place, and precautionary measures should be advised.

SELECTED REFERENCE

Webster, B. H. 1958. Human infection with *Giardia lamblia.* An analysis of 32 cases. *Amer. J. Digest. Dis., 3:* 64.

Dientamebiasis. Although there are a few nonpathogenic amebae that may occur in the human gut, *Dientamoeba fragilis* has often been associated with symptoms that disappear after drug administration. This small ameba lives in the large bowel and may be associated with chronic mushy stools, diarrhea and gastrointestinal disorders such as nausea and vomiting.

Since no cyst stage is known for the organism, a patient presumably becomes infected by ingesting the trophozoite or vegatative stage in food or drink. This stage must be resistant to gastric juice and other intestinal media before setting up an infection site in the large intestine.

Diagnosis depends on a fecal smear from a patient and is based on the microscopic identification of the trophozoite. The stained trophozoite (Fig. 38) usually has two nuclei, the karyosome of which is in clumps. There is no peripheral chromatin, and occasionally the cytoplasm may contain erythrocytes.

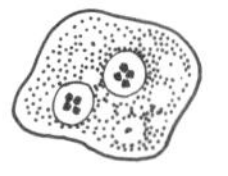

FIG. 38. *Dientamoeba fragilis* trophozoite

It is probably a good idea to routinely treat dientamebiasis cases, especially if a patient has some symptomatology or even chronic mushy stools. Choice and administration of drug is the same as for a case of intestinal amebiasis.

SELECTED REFERENCE

Burrows, R. B., Swerdlow, M. A., Frost, J. K., and Leeper, C. K. 1954. Pathology of *Dientameba fragilis* infections of the appendix. *Amer. J. Trop. Med. & Hyg., 3:* 1033.

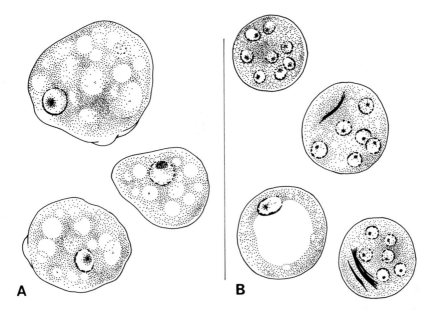

FIG. 39. *Entamoeba coli:* (A) trophozoites; (B) cysts, two of which have chromatoidal bodies.

Other Amebae. There are three other amebae which are not infrequently found in the large intestine of man, and although there is no strong case against them with regard to pathogenesis, they do require differential diagnosis from pathogenic species. The presence of any of these species in a patient indicates that fecal contamination has taken place.

The three species are *Entamoeba coli, Endolimax nana,* and *Iodamoeba bütschlii,* and they all have both trophozoite and cyst stages.

E. coli is more similar to *E. histolytica* than the other two species. The nuclear structure of *E. coli* (whether in a trophozoite or cyst stage) resembles *E. histolytica* in that peripheral chromatin is present, but it is made up of large clumps and is usually heavier on a side (Fig. 39A). Moreover, the single karyosome is larger and usually eccentrically located. The cytoplasm of *E. coli* is more "bumpy" in appearance than the granular nature of *E. histolytica* and rarely includes erythrocytes. In the cyst stage *E. coli* has 8 nuclei in a mature cyst, and in less mature cysts the chromatoidal bodies have splintered ends (Fig. 39B), rather than rounded ends as in *E. histolytica.*

Endolimax is characterized by lacking peripheral chromatin in the nucleus, but rather has a large karyosome (Fig. 40A). There are 4 such nuclei in its mature, oblong cyst (Fig. 40B).

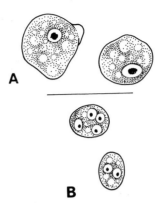

Fɪɢ. 40. *Endolimax nana*: (A) trophozoites; (B) cysts

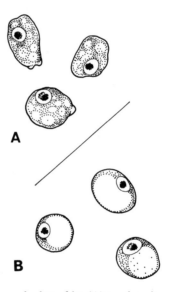

Fɪɢ. 41. *Iodoamoeba bütschlii:* (A) trophozoites; (B) cysts

Iodamoeba also lacks peripheral chromatin in its nucleus but has a large karyosome with acromatic granules piled up on one end of the karyosome (Fig. 41A). The cyst stage has a very prominent glycogen vacuole and usually only 1 nucleus (Fig. 41B).

While it takes considerable study to work up competence to diagnose these amebae with certainty, at least a passing knowledge of their existence serves a purpose of caution in quickly calling an ameba from the intestinal tract as *E. histolytica.*

SELECTED REFERENCE

Brooke, M. M. et al. 1964. Amebiasis: Laboratory Diagnosis. *Public Hlth. Serv. Publ. No. 1184.* Introduction and Parts I, II and III.

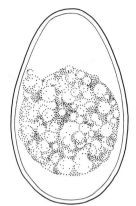

FIG. 42. *Isosporoa* oöcyst

Isoporiasis. There are two species of coccidia of the human intestinal tract, and although they are cosmopolitan in geographic distribution, they are more prevalent in warmer climates. Human *Isospora* probably behave like other coccidia and invade the mucosa lining of the intestinal tract in which various stages of their life cycle take place. Although many human cases are without symptoms, some patients exhibit various degrees of gastrointestinal upset and distress.

A patient acquires the infection by ingesting in food, drink, or in a hand-to-mouth manner the infective oöcysts released in the feces of an infected person. The oocysts are fairly transparent, elongate to oval in shape (Fig. 42) and may contain infective divisional stages of the parasite. The microscopic identification of these stages in a fecal sample constitutes diagnosis. Since the infection is self-limiting (a week or two), treatment is usually not thought to be necessary.

SELECTED REFERENCES

Faust, E. C., Giraldo, L. E., Caicedo, G., and Bonfante, R. 1961. Human isosporiosis in the western hemisphere. *Amer. J. Trop. Med. & Hyg., 10:* 343.
Markell, E. K. 1950. Infection with *Isospora hominis:* Report of two cases. *J. Parasitol., 36:* 500.

Balantidiasis. Balantidium coli is a large ciliate of the large intestine of man and hogs and is similar to *E. histolytica* in many respects. The trophozoite is an efficient producer of ulceration of the large bowel, and signs and symptoms of a case of balantidiasis are similar to those of amebiasis. Trophozoites are found in diarrhetic stools and the cyst stage in formed stools. The life cycle is similar to that of *E. histolytica* except that there is no multiplication in the cyst stage.

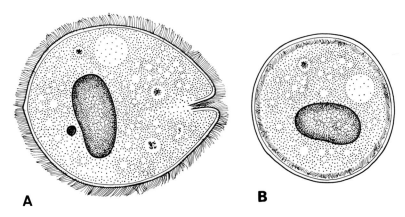

FIG. 43. *Balantidium coli*: (A) trophozoite; (B) cyst

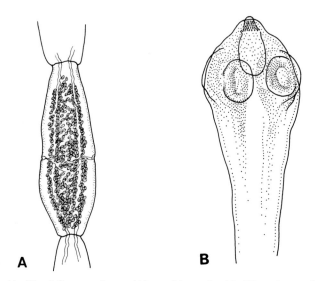

FIG. 44. *Dipylidium caninum*: (A) gravid proglottid; (B) scolex, or head

A patient acquires the infection by fecal contamination of food, drink and fingers. Diagnosis is made by the microscopic identification of the trophozoite and/or cyst stage in a fecal sample. The trophozoite is a huge organism for a protozoan, is covered by rows of cilia, and is very easy to identify (Fig. 43A). The large cyst is subspherical, with a smooth cyst wall and a large, sausage-shaped macronucleus (Fig. 43B). Treatment is by means of diodohydroxyquin and the tetracyclines, as used in intestinal amebiasis.

SELECTED REFERENCES

Arean, V. M., and Koppisch, E. 1956. Balantidiasis. A review and report of cases. *Amer. J. Pathol., 32:* 1089.
Young, M. D. 1939. Balantidiasis. *J.A.M.A., 113:* 580.

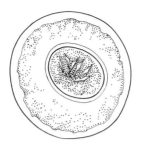

FIG. 45. *Hymenolepis diminuta* egg

Double-barreled Tapeworm. *Dipylidium caninum* is a tapeworm which normally occurs in dogs and cats but occasionally parasitizes man, especially children. An infected patient exhibits gastrointestinal upset and seeks medical advice because of the worm segments observed in the stool.

The worm is acquired by the accidental ingestion of cat or dog fleas containing the larval (*cysticercoid*) stage of the tapeworm. These larvae develop into adulthood in the small intestine. As in beef and pork tapeworm, the segments or proglottids usually detach from the worm proper and either pass out in the feces or migrate to the perianal region.

Diagnosis is based on the morphologic identification of the characteristic proglottids from a stool specimen or from the perianal region. The proglottids have a double set of reproductive organs per segment, and in ripe ones the eggs are grouped in clusters or packets (Fig. 44A). The scolex of the worm is characterized by an introversible proboscis with hooks (Fig. 44B).

Treatment is by quinacrine administration in the manner of other tapeworm infections. Patients should be advised both as to the value of regular deworming of animals and to discourage intimate association of children with pets.

SELECTED REFERENCES

Moore, D. V. 1962. A review of human infections with the common dog tapeworm, *Dipylidium caninum*, in the United States. *The Southwestern Veterinarian, 15:* 283.

Vernard, C. E. 1958. Morphology, binomics, and taxonomy of the cestode *Dipylidium caninum. Ann. N.Y. Acad. Sci., 37:* 273.

Rat Tapeworm. There are vague intestinal symptoms associated with the occasional infection of patients with the rodent tapeworm, *Hymenolepis diminuta*. Infection is obtained by the accidental ingestion of various insects in flour. These arthropods become infected by eating rat droppings harboring tapeworm eggs. Diagnosis is based on the microscopic identification of the characteristic egg in a fecal sample. The egg is subspherical, has a 6-hooked embryo inside, but lacks the polar filaments present in the egg of the dwarf tapeworm (Fig. 45). Treatment is with quinacrine, as with other intestinal tapeworm infections.

SELECTED REFERENCE

Riley, W. A., and Shannon, W. R. 1922. The rat tapeworm, *Hymenolepis diminuta* in man. *J. Parasitol., 8:* 109.

chapter four

GENITOURINARY PARASITES

With two exceptions, the genitourinary system is not a frequent site of parasitism. There has been a variety of protozoan and worm infections reported from the genitourinary tract, but either these are ectopic locations of human pathogens or are primary sites of parasites which rarely occur in man. The two exceptions are the flagellated protozoa responsible for trichomoniasis and the fluke responsible for urinary schistosomiasis. Although the latter parasite is actually an inhabitant of the vascular system (around the urinary bladder), it has a profound effect on the urinary system and will therefore be considered in this chapter.

TRICHOMONIASIS

Trichomonal vaginitis   *Trichomonas vaginalis*

Clinical Picture. There is a varied symptomatology associated with the infection of the genitourinary tract of human males and females with this flagellated protozoan. The male patient is usually asymptomatic but may exhibit urethritis and burning sensations on urination. Some female patients show few symptoms (except during stress periods), whereas in others trichomoniasis can be quite serious. The cardinal sign is vaginal discharge in the form of leukorrhea, accompanied by vaginal itching and burning. There is increased frequency of urination, and the vaginal mucosa may be hyperemic.

Life Cycle. Although the infection is transmitted mostly by the venereal route, this is apparently not the only manner of infection. Vaginal contamination from toilet seats, the water of toilet bowls, and

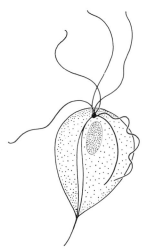

FIG. 46. *Trichomonas vaginalis* trophozoite

from fomites have been indicated. Moreover, there have been cases of young virgins and babies infected with this flagellate.

There is no cyst stage of the flagellate, so transmission simply involves the transfer of the vegetative *trophozoite* stage of the organism from one patient to another by the modes described. There are no animal reservoirs, and the geographic distribution is world-wide.

Diagnosis. The microscopic identification of the organism establishes the diagnosis. In a female patient the sample is taken either from a vaginal discharge or from a genitourinary swab. In a male patient the organism may be recovered either from urethral discharge or from centrifuged urine. The parasite is easily recognized in wet preparations by its jerky motions, an undulating membrane, and a tapered, trailing rod which projects from the posterior end of the animal (Fig. 46).

Treatment. The course of action combines specific chemotherapy and returning the vagina to its normal status. The drug of choice seems to be the oral administration of metronidazole. With female patients this compound is also given concomitantly as vaginal inserts, and acid douches are used as an adjunct to chemotherapy. Even though only husband or wife may be infected, it is important that both undergo chemotherapy at the same time.

Post-Treatment Advice. The only practical counsel is to stress good feminine and male hygiene.

SELECTED REFERENCES

Trussell, R. E. 1947. *Trichomonas vaginalis and Trichomoniasis.* 277 pp., Charles C. Thomas, Springfield, Illinois.

Watt, L. 1965. *Trichomoniasis. The Practitioner, 195:* 613.
Young, R. V. 1949. Trichonomiasis in the male. *Rocky Mt. Med. J., 24:* 928.

URINARY SCHISTOSOMIASIS

Urinary bilharziasis   *Schistosoma haematobium*

Clinical Picture. The effects of the urinary type of schistosomiasis also depend on the factors described for the intestinal type of infection. Bloody urine is an early sign of infection, and in cases of long duration or multiple exposures, scarification and fibrosis of tissue may occur. The bladder loses its elasticity, and constriction, polyp formation and even carcinoma are associated with this infection. Increase in frequency and pain during urination is usual. Pseudotubercle formation in the lungs is also an associated condition of urinary schistosomiasis, since eggs are easily carried to this organ when laid directly in the blood flow of the vesicle plexus.

Life Cycle. The acquisition of infection, migration and maturation of the worms in the body and the life cycle of the trematode inside the snail are similar to that described in intestinal schistosomiasis. The difference is that in addition to some worms being present in the inferior mesenteric network, most are found in the veins of the urinary bladder. Human urinary schistosomiasis is endemic in Africa, the Middle and Near East, with pockets in Portugal and India. Although the human species is naturally present in some other animals, reservoirs of infection are thought not to be important in transmission.

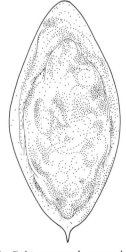

FIG. 47. *Schistosoma haematobium* egg

Diagnosis. The microscopic identification of the *Schistosoma haematobium* egg is diagnostic. The sample is taken from sediment of a urine sample or from centrifuged urine. In chronic cases where eggs are scarce, hatching techniques may be used. The egg is ovoid and has a conspicuous terminal spine (Fig. 47). A fully-developed miracidium is contained within. Since the worms also locate in rectal veins, rectal snips or even stool examinations can also provide diagnosis.

Treatment. Stibophen and lucanthone hydrochloride are the drugs usually administered in urinary schistosomiasis.

Post-Treatment Advice. Preventive measures are the same as for intestinal schistosomiasis. Bronchial symptoms are not unusual after treatment, and this is felt to be associated with the drifting of adult worms into the lungs following a course of chemotherapy.

SELECTED REFERENCES

Azar, J. E., Schaibman, I. G., and Pitchford, R. J. 1958. Some observations on *Schistosoma haematobium* in the human rectum and sigmoid. *Trans. Roy. Soc. Trop. Med. & Hyg., 52:* 562.

Forsyth, D. M. 1965. Treatment of urinary schistosomiasis. Practice and theory. *Lancet, 2:* 354.

Fripp, P. J. 1965. Bilharziasis and bladder cancer. *Brit. J. Cancer, 19:* 292.

chapter five

TISSUE PARASITES

What will be considered as tissue parasites is a heterogeneous collection of organisms which do not cause primary injury to the human integument (excepting *E. histolytica*) and subcutaneous areas of the body, are not parasites of the intestinal or genitourinary tracts, and are not usually diagnosed by blood film examination. These tissue parasites have a common feature of affecting some deeper organ (other than the gut) such as the liver, lungs and central nervous system. Many of these tissue parasites also have the features that they are difficult to diagnose and to treat. Moreover, certain of them are of the most serious of all parasitic infections.

LIVER AMEBIASIS

Entamoeba histolytica

Clinical Picture. Although any organ of the body may become involved with amebic abscesses, by far the most frequent site is the liver. A patient in the early stages of liver infection apparently shows very little, if any, signs or symptoms of disease. As the abscess develops, however, the patient exhibits fever, chills and sweats, and the liver becomes tender and painful—especially on the right side. With the development of a larger ulcer, there is liver enlargement, weight loss, and the pain extends to the right shoulder.

Life Cycle. Although liver abscesses must certainly always develop secondarily from a primary site of infection in the large intestine, many patients with liver involvement have had no history of overt cases of intestinal amebiasis. This points out the potential seriousness of intestinal amebiasis, whether it be acute, subacute, or even in the carrier state. Such patients always run the risk of developing metastatic abscesses in extraintestinal sites.

The trophozoites of *E. histolytica* in the large bowel get into the venules and are carried by the portal veins to the intrahepatic capillaries of the liver. Here they multiply, colonize and begin to cytolyze liver cells. There may be single or multiple lesions which then coalesce into a large abscess. As the abscess increases in size, the center gets necrotic and is filled with a thick, pasty, chocolate-reddish brown material. This material is usually sterile for bacteria and amebae, but amebic trophozoites are located in the peripheral margin of healthy liver tissue. The ulcer may break through to the diaphragm or even into the lung cavity.

Diagnosis. The microscopic identification of the amebic trophozoite from the liver abscess would establish diagnosis, but this is easier said than done. The amount of material that is surgically drained from an abscess and submitted to the diagnostic laboratory is about a quart or so, and the chances of finding amebae in this are about nil. In the final portions of drainage which contain healthy, reddish liver tissue, however, the chances of recovering amebae—either by direct examination or by culture methods—are considerably better. Perhaps the best indirect method of diagnosis is when the patient responds to antiamebic chemotherapy.

Treatment. Emetine and chloroquine are very good drugs against liver amebiasis. Although emetine is the more active of the two compounds, because of its high relative toxicity it is probably best to administer treatment with the less toxic chloroquine. Since the action of chloroquine against possible intestinal amebiasis in the patient is minimal, chemotherapeutic measures should also be directed toward intestinal infection by the use of other drugs, such as diodohydroxyquin.

Post-Treatment Advice. Preventive measures as described for intestinal amebiasis also apply to liver amebiasis. Moreover, the patient's interest should also be directed toward treatment of intestinal amebiasis, which he may have in nonclinical form.

SELECTED REFERENCES

Conal, N. J., Jr. 1949. The treatment of hepatic amebiasis. *Amer. J. Med., 6:* 309.
Shaffer, J. G., Shales, W. H., and Radke, R. A. 1965. *Amebiasis: A Biomedical Problem,* 172 pp., Charles C Thomas, Springfield, Illinois.

TOXOPLASMOSIS

Toxoplasma gondii

Clinical Picture. The effects of toxoplasmosis are protean and depend mostly on whether the patient becomes infected in utero or at some time after birth. In most adults the infection is subclinical, except that in recent years there have been reports that many adults have chorioretinitis and uveitis associated with toxoplasmosis of the eye. In older children the protozoan parasites infect cells of various visceral organs, and the clinical picture includes rash, fever, mental disturbances, extreme fatigue and aches, and atypical pneumonia. The organisms infect various reticuloendothelial cells, leucocytes and parenchymal cells.

If a mother having her first child is infected early in pregnancy, she shows few (if any) symptoms, but the child is usually born with numerous defects. A variety of things may be wrong, but those having the highest frequency are chorioretinitis, cerebral calcification, psychomotor disorders, and hydro- or microcephaly. These conditions in a newborn are most often fatal, but some children linger for some time as irreversible invalids. There is also evidence that some children (although they become infected congenitally) do not show symptoms at birth, but rather some time later exhibit signs of visceral infection —such as liver and splenic enlargement.

Life Cycle. Other than congenital and accidental laboratory infections, nothing is definitely known about the natural life cycle of this parasite. There is every evidence that not only up to 50 % of humans have or have had the infection, but also practically every type of land vertebrate carries the organism in all parts of the world. *Toxoplasma* apparently is a well-adapted parasite, because in most cases these are not apparent infections. Experimentally, the parasite will infect laboratory animals by any route of administration.

Diagnosis. Overt infection in the newborn is suspected by the classical signs and symptoms already described. Definite diagnosis can be made only by laboratory means in which the organisms are microscopically identified. The parasites exist in the proliferative form (acute infection) and in a cyst form (chronic infection).

The proliferative forms are crescent-shaped, usually rounded at one end, and with a single, large nucleus (Fig. 48A). These forms may exist singly or in clusters within fixed cells of the RE system, parenchyma cells of most organs, and in wandering macrophages, blood elements, body fluids, and various exudates. These proliferative organisms can also be microscopically identified from stained peritoneal exudates of laboratory mice which have been intraperitoneally injected with diagnostic samples taken from a patient. Such inoculated mice come down with a generalized infection and die within about a week, and there are masses of parasites in the exudate of their peritoneal cavity.

The cyst form is identified from stained sections and consists of a

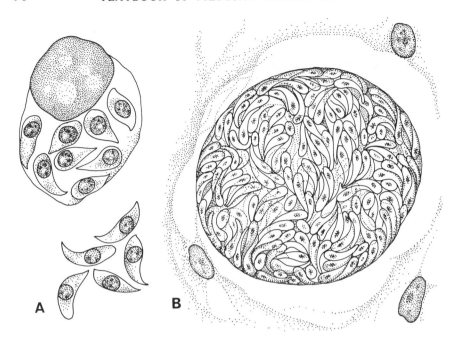

FIG. 48. *Toxoplasma gondii:* (A) proliferative forms of parasite within and free of a macrophage; (B) cyst form from section of brain.

spherical structure having a peripheral membrane and with many organisms inside (Fig. 48B). There is no tissue reaction around the cysts, and they frequently locate in the central nervous system and lungs.

There are several serologic tests, the best of which seems to be the dye test. The basis for this test is that when the organisms harvested from mice are exposed to human serum having *Toxoplasma* antibody (at a pH of 11), the organisms lose their ability to stain with methylene blue. This test indicates past or present infection with the parasite and probably remains positive throughout life. High or rising titers indicate active infection, and negativity rules out toxoplasmosis in the patient.

Treatment. The only known treatment for acute infections is a combination of pyrimethamine and triple sulfonamides. Steroid administration has also been reported to be effective in eye conditions of adults.

Post-Treatment Advice. The question always comes up from parents who have had an overtly infected newborn as to whether future children run the risk of congenital infection. They should be convinced that subsequent children will be protected from infection, since the mother carries antibodies against the parasites. Since the mode(s) of transmission of the parasite remain unknown, there is little advice one can give relative to prevention of infection, except to discourage intimate contact with pets and other animals.

SELECTED REFERENCES

Beattie, C. P. 1963. Toxoplasmosis. *The Practitioner, 191:* 599.
—— 1964. *Toxoplasmosis* (Booklet). 64 pp., The Royal College of Physicians, Edinburgh, Scotland.
Eyles, D. E., Gibson, C. L., Coleman, A. B., and Jones, F. E. 1957. Laboratory aids in the diagnosis of toxoplasmosis. *J. Tenn. State Med. Assoc., 50:* 408.
Frenkel, J. K. 1949. Pathogenesis, diagnosis, and treatment of human toxoplasmosis. *J.A.M.A., 140:* 369.
Remington, J. S., Jacobs, L., and Kaufman, H. E. 1960. Toxoplasmosis in the adult. *New England J. Med., 262:* 180 and 237.
Siim, J. C. (Ed.) 1960. *Human Toxoplasmosis.* 220 pp., The Williams & Wilkins Company, Baltimore.

PARAGONIMIASIS

Oriental lung fluke *Paragonimus westermani*

Clinical Picture. This adult human fluke is normally encapsulated in lung parenchyma, where it causes ulceration and necrosis. Depending on the number of worms, a patient may exhibit degrees of bronchopneumonial or tuberculoid symptoms in which there is cough, chest pain, and malaise. Considerable eosinophilia is usually a feature of the infection. There may be additional signs and symptoms due to ectopic locations of the worms and their eggs in the body. Oftentimes, the liver, muscles and testes are involved, and if the worms locate in the central nervous system, epileptoid seizures may result.

Life Cycle. A patient becomes infected by eating fresh-water crab or crayfish harboring the viable *metacercarial* cysts of the parasite. These infective forms excyst in the small intestine, and the immature worms penetrate the gut and enter the abdominal wall for further development. Following this sojourn, the worms re-enter the abdominal cavity and (via several penetrational paths) reach the pleural cavities and penetrate lung tissue. This route takes a few weeks, and after reaching the lungs, the worms mature to adults in a month or so.

The worms commence egg-laying in their cystic craters, and when these erupt, the fluke eggs are coughed to the sputum of the patient. Most eggs are swallowed, pass through the intestinal tract, and are voided with the feces. The trematode eggs are nonembryonated when leaving the patient and require development in water for a few weeks before a miracidial stage of the parasite develops within.

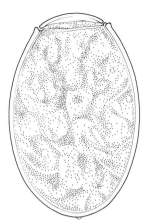

FIG. 49. *Paragonimus westermani* egg

Eventually, the miracidium hatches from the egg, swims about in the water, and penetrates a suitable snail host. Considerable larval multiplication occurs in the snail, and after a few months many cercarial organisms are liberated into the water from infected snails. These cercariae penetrate and encyst in the tissues of certain crabs and crayfish. The parasitic cyst in the crustacean is called the metacercaria and is in the infective stage when man inadvertently eats it. The same or similar species of trematode occurs in man and many other animals (such as the pig, dog, cat, and many felines and rodents), but human infection is geographically located mostly in the Far East, Africa, and possibly South America.

Diagnosis. The microscopic identification of the fluke egg from a stool sample constitutes diagnosis. The egg is similar to that of *D. latum* in morphology, being ovoid in shape, having an operculum (or lid), and a small protuberance at the posterior end. However, differential diagnosis can be made by the fact that the *Paragonimus* egg is more pointed at the end, and the operculum has a "sunken" appearance (Fig. 49). Rusty sputum, pulmonary symptoms and eosinophilia in patients traveling to endemic areas should suggest lung fluke infection. An intradermal skin test is of less value but may assist in diagnosis in cases suspected of having ectopic worms.

Treatment. Until recently there were no highly effective drugs against paragonimiasis. A variety of compounds (such as chloroquine or emetine—alone or in combination) produce symptomatic relief but do not effect cure. The drug of choice now seems to be bithionol.

Post-Treatment Advice. Caution should be advised in the consumption of uncooked crab or crayfish dishes in endemic areas. Curative treatment should also be stressed to prevent ectopic infections.

SELECTED REFERENCES

Yokagawa, M. et al. 1963. Chemotherapy of paragonimiasis with bithionol. V. Studies on the minimum effective dose and changes in abnormal X-ray shadows in the chest after treatment. *Amer. J. Trop. Med. & Hyg., 12:* 859.

Yokagawa, S., Cort, W. W., and Yokagawa, M. 1960. Paragonimus and paragonimiasis. *Exp. Parasitol., 10:* 81 and 139.

CLONORCHIASIS

Chinese liver fluke   *Clonorchis sinensis*

Clinical Picture. The signs and symptoms of a patient infected with Chinese liver fluke vary according to the number of worms present and the degree of liver damage. With few worms there is little or no difficulty. As the worm burden increases, the trematodes cause mechanical and toxic irritation to the biliary radicles in which they usually reside. This results in proliferation and hyperplasia of the bile duct epithelium, leading to blockage and pressure necrosis. The patient may exhibit jaundice, liver enlargement, gastrointestinal upset, and abdominal pain. Eosinophilia is commonly present.

Life Cycle. Infection is acquired by ingestion of viable metacercarial cysts in certain fresh-water fish. The trematodes excyst in the small intestine and eventually reach and mature into adult worms in the biliary radicles in about a month. Eggs released from the flukes pass down into the gut and are voided from the body in the fecal mass.

Clonorchis eggs are very small, and although they have a fully-developed miracidium when passed in the feces, they do not hatch when reaching water. Rather, the eggs must be eaten by a suitable snail host in which generations of larval organisms develop. As is true with all human fluke species, the cercariae eventually develop and are released from the snail into the water.

In this life cycle, the cercariae must penetrate and encyst in the muscles and subcutaneous areas of suitable fish for the metacercarial stage to occur. These infective cysts are infective when a patient eats raw or improperly cooked fish. Clonorchiasis occurs in man and several other animals (cat, dog, pig and several feral animals) in many countries of the Far East.

Diagnosis. The microscopic identification of the egg from a stool sample is the basis for diagnosis. The egg is morphologically similar to the egg of human intestinal heterophyid flukes, but a distinction can be made. The eggs of Clonorchis (Fig. 50) are more pyriform than heterophyid eggs, have a more prominent operculum and an

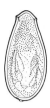

Fig. 50. *Clonorchis sinensis* egg

aboperular, knob-like structure. A further distinction is that the *Clonorchis* egg has a distinct "shouldering" at the opercular end, a feature lacking in the heterophyid eggs.

Hepatic symptoms in a patient from endemic areas should always suggest clonorchiasis. Since the worms live up to 20 years in the body, such consideration should also be made in patients who have been out of endemic areas for many years.

There are two additional closely related species of liver fluke (in the Far East and eastern Europe), but since the eggs and treatment are similar, the distinction need not be made on practical grounds.

Treatment. There is no satisfactory treatment for clonorchiasis, but chloroquine administration seems to result in clinical improvement.

Post-Treatment Advice. The importance of eating only adequately cooked fish from endemic areas should be stressed.

SELECTED REFERENCES

Edelman, M. H., and Spingarn, C. L. 1949. Clonorchiasis in the United States. *J.A. M.A., 140:* 1147.

Ehrenworth, K., and Daniels, R. A. 1958. Clonorchiasis sinensis. Clinical manifestations and diagnosis. *Ann. Int. Med., 49:* 419.

Strauss, W. G. 1962. Clonorchiasis in San Francisco. *J.A.M.A., 179:* 130.

CYSTICERCOSIS

Pork bladder worm   *Taenia solium*

Clinical Picture. Depending mostly on location of the larvae in tissue, cysticercosis, or infection with the bladder worm of the pork tapeworm (*Taenia solium*), results in protean signs and symptoms. Pressure symptoms of various sorts are the rule, but in some cases there may be little or no clinical effects unless the bladder worms are located in a critical area. Cysts in subcutaneous areas and in muscles provoke infiltration of leucocytes, and in time this leads to fibrosis, necrosis, and eventual calcification of the larvae.

The two most critical areas where the cysts may locate are in the brain and the eye. In both these locations there is no fibrous encapsulation of the tapeworm larva. Infection of the eye is usually in the vitreous humor. The most dramatic site of infection is the brain, the effects of which may be headache, nausea, vomiting, and progressive neurologic and epileptoid reactions.

Life Cycle. Although a patient acquires an intestinal infection of adult tapeworm by eating viable bladder worms in hog tissue, the mode of ending up with cysticercosis is quite different—and may happen in either of two ways. In either case, however, the tapeworm eggs hatch in the intestinal tract, the embryo (or oncosphere) penetrates the intestinal wall, gets into the vascular system, and filters out in various parts of the body.

One method of contracting the infection is when a patient swallows the worm eggs containing viable embryos. These eggs may be in food contaminated with the feces of other infected persons or from an intestinal infection of the patient himself. Ingestion of eggs may also take place in a hand-to-mouth fashion in a patient having an intestinal infection.

The other mode of infection is when worm eggs in a patient having an intestinal infection are caused to go forward in the intestinal tract to the level of the duodenum or stomach. This may occur during bouts of vomiting or reverse peristalsis in the gut. Whatever the mode of arrival in the upper intestinal tract, the eggs hatch—and finally end up in various locations of the body as bladder worms.

Essentially what happens in cysticercosis is that man substitutes for the hog in the life cycle. The infection is present in those parts of the world in which public health standards are low and in which adult pork tapeworm infection occurs.

Diagnosis. The only specific means of diagnosis is by the morphologic identification of the tapeworm larva—either excised in toto or from sectioned material. This presents no problems when the cysts are located subcutaneously but is difficult when the bladder worms are in deeper tissue and critical locations.

Once bladder worms undergo calcification, radiographs are useful in their detection. Cysticerci in the eye can be observed by ophthalmologic examination. If one suspects cerebral cysticercosis, it may be helpful in diagnosis to examine other body areas for bladder worms before operative measures are taken. Although almost all cases of cysticercosis involve pork tapeworm, there have been a few cases due to bladder worms of the beef tapeworm, *T. saginata.*

The bladder worms are elongate or pea-shaped, and grossly visible (Fig. 51B). They are filled with fluid (Fig. 51A) and have a dense area on one side. It is this dense area that contains the head, or scolex, of the tapeworm. In the pork tapeworm there is a crown of

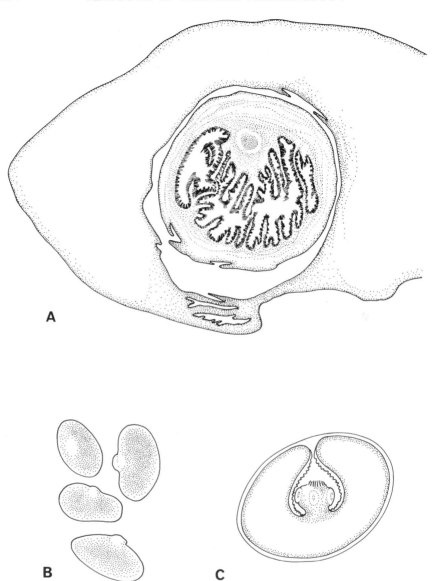

Fig. 51. *Taenia solium:* (A) section through cysticercus, or bladder worm; (B) bladder worms, entire, excised from tissue; (C) section of a single cysticercus larva.

hooks on the scolex (Fig. 51C), whereas these hooks are lacking in the beef tapeworm larva.

Treatment. There is no effective chemotherapy for cysticercosis, and the only course of action is surgical removal of the bladder worms. The benefit and risk of surgery depends on the number of larval worms, their location in the body, and the clinical judgment of the physician.

Post-Treatment Advice. The same preventive comments given for adult pork tapeworm infection apply to cysticercosis. Since the tapeworm egg is immediately infective, all persons involved in the diagnosis and treatment of intestinal pork tapeworm infection should be cautioned as to the importance of personal hygiene, and proper precautions ought to be taken in the handling of materials related to the case.

SELECTED REFERENCES

Bickerstaff, E. R. 1955. Cerebral cysticercosis; common but unfamiliar manifestations. *Brit. Med. J., 1:* 1055.

Dixon, H. B. F., and Lipscomb, F. M. 1961. Cysticercosis—An analysis and follow-up of 450 cases. *Privy Council, Med. Res. Special Rep., Ser. No. 299*, 58 pp., London.

Vakil, V. V., and Sirsat, M. V. 1965. Cysticercosis in man. *Indian J. Med. Sci., 19:* 667.

HYDATID DISEASE

Unilocular hydatid cyst   *Echinococcus granulosus*

Alveolar hydatid cyst   *Echinococcus multilocularis*

Clinical Picture. The signs and symptoms of this larval tapeworm infection vary according to which of two types of the infection a patient has, how old the infection is, and what part of the body is involved. The human liver is the focus of infection in most cases, although the lungs, kidneys and even bone may be infected.

Hydatid disease has some characteristics of a developing tumor. Although mechanical and toxic injury results to the organs affected, there are usually no symptoms during the early phase of infection. Eventually there is abdominal pain, vomiting, pressure symptoms, and necrosis to the invaded tissue. If fluid seeps from the sac of tapeworm larvae, systemic toxicity in the patient usually results. There is considerable eosinophilia, and the seepage of fluid may result in fatal hypersensitivity.

Life Cycle. A patient becomes infected accidentally by ingesting tapeworm eggs, and as in cysticercosis, man actually substitutes for the usual intermediate host. There are two species of tapeworm responsible for hydatid infections.

One of them, *Echinococcus granulosis,* is a very small tapeworm that usually lives in the intestine of dogs. The worm eggs are passed in the feces of infected canines and are accidentally eaten by such animals as grazing sheep and man. These eggs hatch in the small intestine, and the embryo, or oncosphere, penetrates the gut, gets into the vascular system, and then filters out mostly in the liver and lungs.

Whether in man or sheep, in these organs there develops a vacu-

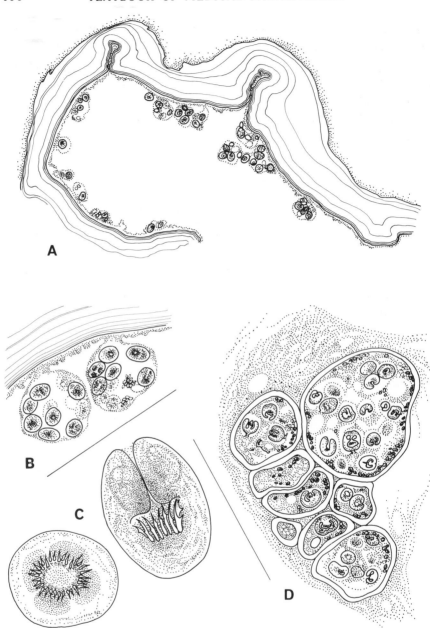

Fig. 52. Hydatid cysts: (A) section through a portion of a unilocular cyst; (B) enlarged view of a segment of a unilocular cyst; (C) surface and sectional views of a single echinococcus larva; (D) section through an alveolar cyst.

olated larval stage, the *hydatid* cyst, or *echinococcus* larva. Initially, it is very small (about 1 cm), and its subsequent development is very slow. There is extensive multiplication of new worm larvae from the inner germinative layer of the cyst. The outer layer of the cyst is made up of host tissue encapsulation. Eventually, a large, unilocular cyst is developed which contains much fluid inside (up to 2 quarts have been removed from a single hydatid). Although most cysts contain thousands of larvae (*hydatid sand*) (Fig. 52A) some cysts may be sterile (with respect to tapeworm larvae) because of bacterial contamination. If bone is infected by a hydatid, there is little outer encapsulation, but rather an extension of the cyst into the bone canals. This results in considerable osseous erosion.

The other species, *Echinococcus multilocularis*, has a carnivore-rodent life cycle in nature. Foxes are usually the hosts for the adult tapeworm, and field rodents and man are infected with the echinococcus larva. Infections of man and rodents result from ingestion of the tapeworm eggs, and the general life cycle is similar to that of *E. granulosus*. The primary sites of infection in man are the liver and lungs, but—unlike the unilocular type—there is no definite tissue encapsulation or limiting membrane around the tapeworm larva. Growth and development of additional larvae is by exogenous budding (Fig. 52D), rather than by the endogenous mode as occurs in *E. granulosus*. In time there is such progressive invasion of the infected area that the tissue becomes honeycombed. The center of the developing cyst breaks down into an abscess, while the peripheral part of the cyst continues to grow and multiply into adjacent tissue areas. There is no fluid formed as in the unilocular type of hydatid, but rather the ground substance is a gelatinous material. In many ways, this alveolar or multilocular hydatid behaves as a neoplasm.

In both types of hydatid the patient is a blind end to the infection cycle. In nature the infected tissues of rodents and sheep must be eaten for continuation of the life cycle.

Diagnosis. The only definite means of diagnosis is by the microscopic identification of the tapeworm scolex, or head, from aspirates of the cyst. The scolex has muscular sucking discs and a crown of hooks (Figs. 52B & 52C). It should be emphasized that the procedure of aspiration is risky in that it may induce hypersensitive reactions in the patient. Consequently, it is not widely used.

Early asymptomatic cases are usually discovered by radiographs made for some other reason. Other diagnostic methods include a skin test. If positive, it indicates that the patient has or has had hydatid infection; if negative, it rules out infection with hydatid. Various serologic tests have also been used in establishing presumptive diagnosis.

Hydatids should be suspected in any cystic tumor not otherwise explained. Unilocular infection is cosmopolitan in geographic distribution and is most prevalent in the great sheep-raising districts of the world. Alveolar infections are also widespread but most prevalent in Central and Eastern Europe.

Treatment. Surgery is the only means of treatment in hydatid cases. Since this involves the risk of inducing anaphylactoid reactions in the patient, after surgical exposure of the cyst fluid is aspirated and replaced with 10 % formalin before removing the cyst.

Many late cases (especially of the alveolar type) are inoperable by the time diagnosis has been established. In such cases the only course of action is the injection of sterile hydatic fluid antigens (so-called biotherapy), with the hope of death of the cyst and its eventual absorption.

Post-Treatment Advice. The potential danger of close association with dogs should always be emphasized, as well as the risk of eating raw, wild fruit.

SELECTED REFERENCES

Cahill, K. M. 1963. Echinococcosis. *New York M. Med., 63:* 1964.

Cameron, T. W. M., and Webster, G. 1961. The ecology of hydatidosis. IN *Studies in Disease Ecology,* J. M. May, Ed. 11. 141–160. Hafner Publishing Company, Inc., New York.

Hargreaves, W. H. 1963. Hydatid disease. *The Practitioner, 191:* 615.

Katz, A. M., and Pan, C. 1958. *Echinococcus* disease in the United States. *Amer. J. Med., 15:* 759.

La Fond, D. J., Thatcher, D. S., and Handeyside, R. G. 1963. Alveolar hydatid disease. *J.A.M.A., 186:* 35.

TRICHINOSIS

Trichina worm   *Trichinella spiralis*

Clinical Picture. The vast majority of trichinosis cases appear to be asymptomatic. The clinical effects of the infection are protean and depend on the number of larval worms taken into the body, general health and immunity (based on prior exposure of the patient to trichinosis), and location of the parasites in the body. Active cases of trichinosis have been confused with many other diseases, and a list of misdiagnoses is quite impressive. In a few words, however, diarrhea and fever, followed by muscular pains, periorbital edema, and eosinophilia should always suggest infection with this nematode worm.

When symptomatic, a case of trichinosis may be conveniently separated into three stages (associated with the sequential location of the parasites in the body). A few days to a week following infection there is gastrointestinal upset due to inflammation of the small intestine, abdominal pain, diarrhea, fever, nausea, and the beginning of eosinophilia. In a week to a month there may be 50 to 90 % eosinophilia, intense muscular pains, respiratory difficulties, periorbital edema, and splinter hemorrhages under the fingernails. From about a month to some weeks there is exaggeration of the second stage with continued edema of the arms and abdomen, scaling of the skin—and cardiac and neurologic symptoms in severe cases.

In a few words, inflammation, encapsulation, and calcification constitute host reaction to trichina larvae in muscle. Myocarditis and central nervous system involvement are the most serious complications of trichinosis. General pathology results from a combination of mechanical, toxic and allergic factors.

Life Cycle. A patient becomes infected with the causative nematode agent of trichinosis by eating meat containing viable, encysted trichina larvae. Although these larvae exist in a wide variety of animals (pig, rat, seal, bear, man), a patient's acquisition is almost exclusively from eating infected pork. The same animal, whether it be man or otherwise, temporarily harbors the adult worms in the small intestine and the larvae in tissue—specifically, striated muscle. After a patient eats infected meat, the larvae are freed from the meat and in a few days mature into male and female nematodes in the small intestine. The small worms copulate, and shortly thereafter most of the males pass out of the body in the fecal mass.

The female worms, however, deposit active, living larvae in the intestinal mucosa for about six weeks. These larvae get into lymph and blood and travel around in the general circulation. They may end up in any part of the body, but encystment of larvae takes place only if they reach striated muscle. The muscles mostly infected are those of the limbs, tongue, larynx, diaphragm, gastrocnemius, detloid, and the abdominal wall.

Once in striated muscle, the larvae grow, molt and become sexually differentiated. Muscle tissue forms a cyst around the larvae in about 30 days, and eventually calcification takes place in about 6 months to a year. Some cases of trichinosis show thousands of encysted larvae per gram of muscle.

Diagnosis. A basis for suspecting and diagnosing trichinosis is not always an easy task. Patients usually turn themselves in because of muscular pains and periorbital edema. The determination of recent ingestion of pork is important, especially if a family group or other gathering of people becomes sick—and particularly if noncommercial pork or pork products have been recently consumed.

The microscopic identification of the trichina larvae from muscle biopsy establishes definite diagnosis. The biopsy ought to be taken from the most painful muscle area that is easily accessible. The gastrocnemius and deltoid are favorite sites. The material may be digested with artificial gastric juice, sectioned and stained, or simply pressed between glass slides and examined under the microscope for trichina larvae.

Nonencapsulated larvae indicate an infection of only a few weeks. Noncalcified, encapsulated larvae indicate an infection of a few months' duration. Calcified cysts are the result of old infections and are of no immediate significance.

The encapsulated larva (Fig. 53) is coiled on itself and has a barrel-shaped sheath. There are inflammatory and degenerative changes in the surrounding muscle fibers, and pronounced fat globules at the poles. Meganuclei are also common.

Muscle biopsy is of no value during the first three weeks of infection, since the larvae have not penetrated striated muscle at that time.

There is an intradermal skin test which shows a positive skin reaction of the immediate type in about 15 minutes. In infected persons, however, this test does not become positive during the initial 3 to 4 weeks of a primary case. The reaction also remains positive for some years after infection with trichinosis. The real value of this skin test is when a patient shows a negative skin test in the early stages of examination and then a positive one after some weeks. It is also useful, of course, in ruling out trichinosis.

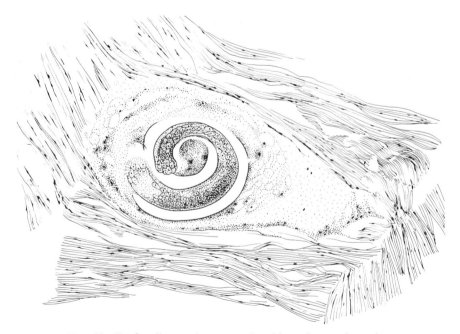

Fig. 53. *Trichinella spiralis*; encapsulated larva in muscle section

There are various other serologic tests, the most widely used being the bentonite slide flocculation test. The material for this test is commercially available and consists of bentonite particles to which *Trichinella* antigen has been adsorbed. Such particles clump very quickly in the presence of serum from a patient containing *Trichinella* antibody. The test is quite specific, and its being negative after 2 weeks' illness of a patient may rule out trichinosis.

Treatment. There is no practical specific chemotherapy for trichinosis, and the outcome of a case depends mostly on how many larvae are eaten and the degree of immunity of a patient prior to infection. There are drugs active against the adult worms in the intestine, but by the time diagnosis is made, these worms are of little importance to the clinical picture. Corticosteroids have been used to treat the inflammatory response in the gut, but this practice is not now in much favor, since it may actually serve to increase the future burden of larvae in tissue. However, steroid treatment does give considerable symptomatic relief in acute cases and (if given early enough) may have value in preventing irreversible neurologic pathology.

The compound thiabendazole has been reported to give relief for muscular pains, but its real value for human trichinosis awaits further testing.

Post-Treatment Advice. The proper cooking of pork and pork products are preventive measures against trichinosis. Deep-freezing of pork kills the larvae but is a much neglected method of control, although practiced unknowingly by many persons who own deep freezers. It should be emphasized that the federal government does not routinely inspect pork for trichina larvae, except when the product is advertised as requiring no further cooking.

SELECTED REFERENCES

Gould, S. E. 1945. *Trichinosis.* 356 pp., Charles C Thomas, Springfield, Illinois.
Maynard, J. E., and Kagan, I. G. 1963. Trichinosis. *The Practitioner, 191:* 622.
Most, H. 1965. Trichinellosis in the United States. *J.A.M.A., 193:* 99.
Spaeth, G. L., Adams, R. E., and Soffe, A. M. 1964. Treatment of trichinosis. *Arch. Ophthalmol., 71:* 359.

VISCERAL LARVA MIGRANS

Dog ascarid   *Toxocara canis*

Cat ascarid   *Toxocara cati*

Clinical Picture. Visceral larva migrans is a clinical syndrome in which nematode larvae of a particular kind set up granulomatous lesions in any part of the body of a patient, but particularly in the liver, lungs, eye and brain.

As in most helminthic infections, signs and symptoms vary according to the number of parasites, their location in the body, and—in this case—according to the degree of hypersensitivity of the patient. The condition is found mostly in children of very young age and is characterized by fever, cough, sundry pains, liver enlargement, persisting hypereosinophilia, dermatitis, and—in severe cases—neurologic signs.

Life Cycle. A patient becomes infected by swallowing worm eggs from soil or from the fur of dogs and cats. These animals are highly infected with an intestinal nematode, *Toxocara* (which has a life cycle similar to the life cycle of *Ascaris* in humans), and which perpetuates itself from dog to dog and from cat to cat.

If a human substitutes for a dog or cat and accidentally ingests the larvated eggs, the larvae hatch in his intestine, penetrate the gut wall and enter the circulatory system. But the larvae do not make the lung-respiratory circuit back to the intestine as mature worms. Instead, they wander into any tissue or organ of the body, inducing inflammatory reactions. This is the end of the road for them (since they are absorbed after several months), but in the interim they are responsible for the difficulties described above.

Diagnosis. The only specific means of diagnosis is by microscopic identification of the nematode larva from a liver biopsy specimen. There are problems connected with this procedure, especially in very young children, and since there is no specific chemotherapy, such a course of action seems radical.

A presumptive diagnosis can be made of a case if there are chronic, nonexplained, pulmonary signs and symptoms, chronic eosinophilia, and liver enlargement. Such a presumption is even more logical if a child has dirt-eating habits, and his pet dog or cat can be shown to have *Toxocara* adult worms in its gut.

Treatment. Since there are no known effective drugs against this nematode larva, the only course of action is symptomatic treatment and supportive measures.

Post-Treatment Advice. Patients and/or parents should be informed that puppies and kittens are more often infected than adult dogs and cats and that a veterinarian should be consulted to establish a regular schedule for deworming these animals. They should also be advised that the family sand box is additional risk in the transmission of this infection.

SELECTED REFERENCES

Beaver, P. C. 1956. Larva migrans. *Exp. Parasitol., 6:* 587.
——— 1962. Toxocariasis (visceral larva migrans) in relation to tropical eosinophilia. *Bull. Soc. Pathol. Exot., 55:* 557.

Brain, L., and Allan, B. 1964. Encephalitis due to infection with *Toxocara canis. Lancet,* *1:* 1355.

Woodruff, A. W., Ashton, N., and Stott, G. J. 1961. *Toxocara canis* infection of the eye. *Trans. Roy. Soc. Trop. Med. & Hyg., 55:* 13.

SUNDRY TISSUE INFECTIONS

Pneumocystic pneumonia *Pneumocystis carinii*
Eosinophilic meningoencephalitis *Angiostrongylus cantonensis*

There has been a variety of other parasites reported from the tissues of man, but (except for the two infections considered below) these are usually natural parasites of animals other than man, and their incidence in people is quite low, and the clinical effects are minor.

Pneumocystic Pneumonia. The condition of interstitial plasma-cell pneumonia occurs mostly in children from a few weeks to several months old. It is characterized by cough, weakness, followed by infiltration of the lungs with plasma cells, and consolidation and congestion of air spaces with fluid. Fever is generally lacking. The condition is highly contagious; it has a propensity for premature babies, and outbreaks in hospitals have occurred. Fatalities may run up to 60%. Associated with this kind of pneumonia is what seems to be a protozoal organism, *Pneumocystis carinii,* of unknown relationship to other organisms. This same organism is also found in a wide variety of domestic animals.

Diagnosis of human cases is difficult and is usually based on post-mortem findings. Touch smears made from the lungs (or tissue that has been sectioned) show cyst-like structures with 1 to 8 nuclei. The life cycle of the organism is unknown, but probably it is transmitted by droplet infection. There is no effective chemotherapy, and treatment is symptomatic and supportive. Human cases should be placed in strict isolation.

SELECTED REFERENCES

Robbins, J. B. et al. 1965. *Pneumocystis carinii* pneumonia. *New England J. Med., 272:* 708.

Watanabe, J. M. et al. 1965. *Pneumocystis carinii* pneumonia in a family. *J.A.M.A., 193:* 685.

Eosinophilic Meningoencephalitis. The clinical effects of this nematode infection in patients of the Far East include fever, headache, stiffness of the neck, and—in some cases—facial paralysis. There is a cerebrospinal fluid pleocytosis consisting of up to 30 % eosinophils. The essential lesion is granulomatous caused by the nematode larvae in the meninges. The disease is usually relatively mild and self-limiting. The causative agent is a nematode, *Angiostrongylus cantonensis,* the adults of which normally reside in the lungs of rats.

The life cycle is such that the larvae develop in land snails and slugs. When these gastropods are eaten, the larvae temporarily reside in the meninges of the rodent and later develop to maturity in the lungs. The method by which patients acquire the infection is not completely settled, but the possible modes are by ingestion of snails, slugs, shrimp-like crustaceans, and possibly other small land invertebrates. The penetration of human skin by the larvae after being emitted from the snail host has also been suggested as a means of infection. Treatment is simply symptomatic and supportive.

SELECTED REFERENCES

Alicata, J. E. 1962. *Angiostrongylus cantonensis* as a causative agent of eosinophilic meningo-encephalitis of man in Hawaii and Tahiti. *Canad. J. Zool., 40:* 5.

Rosen, L. et al. 1962. Eosinophilic meningo-encephalitis caused by a metastrongylid lung-worm of rats. *J.A.M.A., 179:* 620.

chapter six

VASCULAR PARASITES

In terms of the number of human cases of morbidity and mortality, the vascular parasites constitute the major group of parasitic organisms. Although this is an artificial classification of parasites, they do, nevertheless, have several features in common. In a patient each of them usually begins as an infection either free or in some element of the vascular system. Other similarities include the fact that transmission is either directly or indirectly via insect bite, and the chief approach to diagnosis is by means of the stained blood film.

The schistosome worms may also be considered as vascular parasites, but since their effects to a patient so clearly involve the intestinal and urinary systems, they have been considered previously in those respective sections. Moreover, based again on the clinical picture in a patient, Oriental sore and American cutaneous leishmaniasis have been considered as integumentary parasites.

VISCERAL LEISHMANIASIS

Kala-azar   *Leishmania donovani*

Clinical Picture. Although the mode of infection in a patient with visceral leishmaniasis is similar to that of Oriental sore and American cutaneous leishmaniasis, the parasitic flagellates of kala-azar set up a generalized infection of the reticuloendothelial system (especially in the liver, lymph nodes, spleen, bone marrow, and intestine), rather than as integumentary lesions.

The nature of the infection and disease varies in different parts of the world. Consequently, there are no standard signs and symptoms. Generally, a papule may or may not develop at the site of the sandfly

115

bite. The incubation period may take up to several months, during which time there is extensive multiplication of the leishmanial parasites in the macrophage system of the liver, spleen, bone marrow, and intestine. Hyperplasia of the lymphoid-macrophage system results in enlargement, especially of the liver and spleen. An infected patient usually shows varied high fever and other malarial symptoms, as well as weight loss, anemia, extreme diarrhea, and a swollen abdomen. In untreated cases there is extreme emaciation and high mortality, due usually to pneumonic complications.

Life Cycle. The ordinary means of infection is by way of the bite of an infected sandfly containing the leptomonal parasites. However, leishmanial organisms have been recovered from the urine, saliva, feces and tonsils of infected patients, and man-to-man transmission may occur. In certain parts of the world animals other than man play an important role in the transmission of the infection. These include dogs in the Mediterranean area, dogs and cats in South America, and possibly feral animals in the Sudan.

Diagnosis. Since the clinical picture of visceral leishmaniasis may be confused with that of malaria, typhoid fever, and other infections, microscopic identification of the leishmanial organisms is of prime importance. The leishmanial parasites (Fig. 54A) are morphologically identical with those of Oriental sore and American cutaneous leishmaniasis.

There are various approaches to diagnosis. Stained blood films may reveal the leishmanial parasites in monocytes. Blood from a case may also be cultured in vitro for leptomonal organisms (Fig. 54B), and hamsters are very susceptible to experimental infections. When blood films are negative, and for quicker diagnosis, many workers use biopsy methods, the chief of which is sternal bone marrow. The microscopic examination of such stained material is very productive for detecting leishmanial parasites.

Visceral leishmaniasis has wide geographical distribution and is found in most land areas of the world except upper North America and Australia.

Treatment. Immediate relief may be accomplished by the use of antimonials such as ethylstibamide. In cases of antimony resistance or sensitivity, aromatic diamidines such as stilbamidine are indicated. Both of these types of compounds may be quite toxic and require parenteral administration over some weeks.

A dermal leishmanoid rash may develop after treatment and involves the appearance of macules (either depigmented or erythemic) on various area os the body.

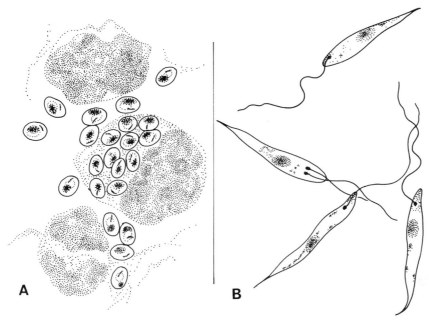

A   B

FIG. 54. *Leishmania donovani:* (A) leishmanial forms of parasite in bone marrow smear; (B) leptomonal forms of parasite from culture.

Post-Treatment Advice. Preventive advice involves the control of sandflies by means of residual DDT spraying of households and by personal repellents. The usual mesh of house screens is not small enough to keep out sandflies.

SELECTED REFERENCES

Manson-Bahr, P. E. C. 1961. Immunity in kala-azar. *Trans. Roy. Soc. Trop. Med. & Hyg., 55:* 550.

Omran, Abdel-Rahim. 1961. The ecology of leishmaniasis. IN *Studies in Disease Ecology,* J. M. May, Ed., pp. 331–388. Hafner Publishing Company, Inc., New York.

AFRICAN TRYPANOSOMIASIS

Mid-African sleeping sickness   *Trypanosoma gambiense*

East African sleeping sickness   *Trypanosoma rhodesiense*

Clinical Picture. There are two clinical types of African trypanosomiasis—caused by two variants of a hemoflagellate protozoan parasite—*Trypanosoma gambiense,* producing a chronic, relatively low virulence syndrome, and *Trypanosoma rhodesiense,* causing a more acute, virulent type of the disease. Both are transmitted by the bite of tsetse flies.

In *T. gambiense* infection the incubation period varies from a few days to several weeks. An initial sign is a nodule at the site of the insect bite. A patient develops irregular fever, headache, and intestinal upset, followed by painful enlargement of lymph nodes, particularly the posterior cervical ones. After several months when the central nervous system becomes involved with the parasites, an infected patient exhibits apathy, lassitude, emaciation, facial swelling, and then progressive motor and sensory changes, leading to mental deterioration and coma.

The clinical picture of *T. rhodesiense* is essentially the same except that the incubation period is much shorter and the sequence of events occurs more rapidly. The patient ususally shows more severe fever and rapid weight loss but less visible involvement of lymph glands. Since patients with *T. rhodesiense* infection usually run a fatal course within a year, the usual signs and symtpoms associated with *T. gambiense* infection are minimal.

Life Cycle. Patients become infected by the bite of tsetse flies. The parasites undergo cyclic development in these insects, and the infective flagellates are inoculated with the insect bite. These flies may also transmit the organisms mechanically from one patient to another during epidemics.

After the trypansomes are introduced into the blood of a patient, they undergo extensive multiplication in the vascular system. During the early phase of the infection the organisms periodically appear and disappear in the blood stream. This is followed by their multiplication interstitially in lymph nodes.

Eventually, the organisms enter the cerebrospinal fluid, producing perivascular infiltration around the capillaries of the central nervous system.

T. gambiense is mostly a man-to-man infection, whereas *T. rhodesiense* transmission involves several large game animals as reservoir hosts. These infections are confined to Africa: *T. gambiense* in Central and Western Africa and *T. rhodesiense* in East Africa.

Diagnosis. The only definite means of diagnosis is by microscopic identification of the organisms. Both clinical variants are morphologically identical on a practical basis. They are very pleomorphic parasites but are generally grouped into slender organisms with a long, free flagellum; short, stumpy forms with little or no free flagellum; and intermediate-sized and shaped parasites. All morphologic types have a prominent nucleus, a granule-like kinetoplast posterior to the nucleus, and a wavy, undulating membrane which runs the length of the body (Fig. 55).

In early cases the hemoflagellates are microscopically identified by

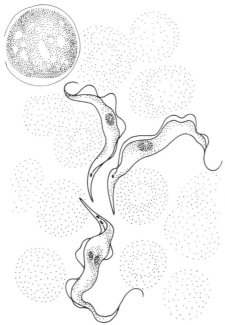

Fɪɢ. 55. *Trypanosoma gambiense* or *rhodesiense;* trypanosomal parasites in blood smear.

stained thin or thick film. Later in the infection, the organisms are more often found in lymph node aspirates, and in late cases it may be necessary to examine cerebrospinal fluid. In either early or late cases the inoculation of diagnostic samples into susceptible laboratory rodents also has value, as microscopic examination of the blood of these rodents after several days will reveal trypanosomes of the same type as in human infection.

Treatment. Suramin and various aromatic diamidines, such as pentamidine, are probably the drugs of choice in early cases. In older infections (where the administration of these drugs does not result in their entering the cerebrospinal fluid) arsenicals such as tryparsamide, mel B, and melarsen oxide are useful. The latter two drugs also have the advantage of being active in the early phase of the infection.

Various nitrofurans have value in central nervous system cases, and such compounds as pentamidine and suramin are useful in chemoprophylaxis of the disease.

All African trypanosomiasis drugs have a relative high toxicity and should be administered with great caution.

Post-Treatment Advice. Persons in endemic areas should be advised of the possibility of chemoprophylaxis.

SELECTED REFERENCES

Duggan, A. J. 1959. An approach to clinical problems of Gambian sleeping sickness. *J. Trop. Med., 62:* 268.

Nash, T. A. M. 1960. A review of the African trypanosomiasis problem. *Trop. Dis. Bull., 57:* 974.

Williamson, J. 1962. Chemotherapy and chemoprophylaxis in Arican trypanosomiasis. *Exp. Parasitol., 12:* 274.

World Health Organization. 1963. Trypanosomiasis. *Bull. Wld. Hlth. Org., 28:* 537.

CHAGAS' DISEASE

American trypanosomiasis   *Trypanosoma cruzi*

Clinical Picture. The clinical effects of American trypanosomiasis, or Chagas' disease, vary according to such factors as age, number of exposures, and duration of infection with the protozoan flagellate.

Although many cases appear to be asymptomatic, the usual acute case begins with a cutaneous granuloma, or "chagoma," at the point where infective parasites were introduced into the skin of a patient. This initial lesion gradually subsides, and after incubation for a period of some days to weeks the patient experiences chills, fever, and muscular pains. Most often there is moderate enlargement of lymph glands and unilateral facial swelling, particularly of the eye (Romaña's sign). Following the acute stage, the parasites multiply in macrophages of such organs as the liver and spleen and also in cardiac muscle and in the microglia cells of the central nervous system. The acute phase is very serious in young infants and often leads to fatality due to nervous involvement.

In chronic cases (especially of long duration) the parasites multiply in various locations throughout the body but seem to have a predilection for cardiac (Fig. 56C) and nervous tissue. There is inflammation and progressive degeneration of affected areas. Heart dilatation and failure, as well as neuropathologic changes, are the usual rule.

Life Cycle. The insect hosts are various members of reduviid bugs, often referred to as cone-nosed, assassin or kissing bugs. The infective flagellates develop in the gut of these insects but are not released to the mouthparts. Rather, a patient is infected by contamination of the bite with the fecal material of the insect released while it is sucking blood from a patient. The infective trypanosomal organisms gain entrance into the wound and are engulfed by macrophages in the developing chagoma.

In the acute phase (especially during the febrile attack) the *trypanosomal* organisms circulate in the blood. As the infection becomes more chronic, the parasites begin to multiply in RE cells of various organs

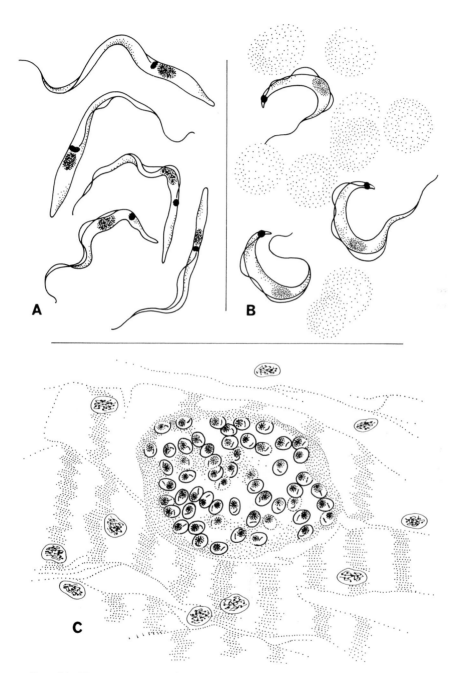

FIG. 56. *Trypanosoma cruzi:* (A) crithidial and trypanosomal forms of parasite from culture; (B) trypanosomal forms in blood smear; (C) cluster of leishmanial forms in section of heart tissue.

and in cells of heart (Fig. 56C) and brain tissue in the *leishmanial* form. Periodically, trypanosomal forms may circulate in the blood (although they do not divide in that medium), but the lasting stage of the parasite in a patient is in fixed cells of the body.

Chagas' disease is found naturally in many animals other than man —dogs and cats, various rodents, and other feral animals. It is distributed widely in South and Central America and is found in certain portions of the United States.

Diagnosis. In the early stages of the infection the trypanosomal forms may be microscopically identified from stained blood films. They may be long and thin or short and stumpy, but all tend to be either U- or C-shaped, having a large kinetoplast at the posterior end of the body (Fig. 56B).

As the trypansomal forms become less numerous in the blood, other approaches to diagnosis are required. Blood or lymph gland biopsy may be cultured in artificial media or injected into suitable laboratory rodents. Positive cases will show living flagellates in vitro (Fig. 56A) or from blood examinations of rodents after several days.

Also used to detect chronic cases is the practice of xenodiagnosis in which laboratory-reared bugs are allowed to feed on a patient. Positive cases will result in the development of infected bugs several days later.

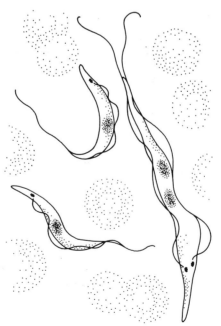

FIG. 57. *Trypanosoma rangeli* in peripheral blood smear.

The complement fixation test has also proved of value in the diagnosis of chronic cases.

T. cruzi must be distinguished from another trypanosome which may infect people—*Trypanosoma rangeli*. The latter organism is non-pathogenic and can be distinguished by its larger size, a smaller kinetoplast, and by the fact that dividing forms occur in peripheral blood smears from patients (Fig. 57).

Treatment. On practical grounds there is no specific chemotherapy against Chagas' disease. There are several compounds active against the early blood phase of the disease, but since this is transient and not often diagnosed, they have limited value. There are no known compounds active against the persisting leishmanial organisms in fixed tissue. Symptomatic and supportive treatment is the only practical course of action at present.

Post-Treatment Advice. Insecticiding of households is the only practical advice one can give.

SELECTED REFERENCES

Massumi, R. A., and Gooch, A. 1965. Chagas' myocarditis. *Arch. Int. Med., 116:* 531.

Noble, E. R. 1955. The morphology and life cycles of trypanosomes. *Quart. Rev. Biol., 30:* 1.

Packchanian, A. A. 1943. Infectivity of the Texas strain of *Trypanosoma cruzi* to man. *Amer. J. Trop. Med., 23:* 309.

Woody, N. C., and Woody, H. B. 1955. American trypanosomiasis (Chagas' Disease). First indigenous case in the United States. *J.A.M.A., 159:* 476.

World Health Organization. 1960. Chagas' Disease. *Tech. Rep. Ser. No. 202.*

MALARIA

Vivax malaria	*Plasmodium vivax*
Falciparum malaria	*Plasmodium falciparum*
Quartan malaria	*Plasmodium malariae*
Ovale malaria	*Plasmodium ovale*

Clinical Picture. Basically, malaria is characterized by periodic chills, fever, and sweating (in that order), and may be accompanied by anemia, splenomegaly, and many other complications—depending on the particular case. This kind of a clinical picture is, of course, found in many other types of infections and is therefore inconstant and hardly specific. Actually, there are four types of malaria (*vivax, ovale, quartan* and *falciparum*), each morphologically distinct in the human and having various other differences in man and in the mosquito which transmits the infection.

The incubation in a patient depends on many factors, among which are the number of sporozoan parasites introduced, the rate of their development in man, and the type of malarial species. Although clinical symptoms do not appear in a patient until the parasites reach a certain density in the blood, the incubation period is shortest in falciparum malaria (7 to 10 days), longest in quartan malaria (about a month), and about 14 days in both vivax and ovale malaria.

In primary cases of vivax and ovale malaria the patient usually experiences headache, muscular pains, and low-grade fever. This is followed by sudden, shaking chills accompanied by peaking fever. During the chilling period, headache and muscular pains are intensified, vomiting is common, and there are respiratory and vascular difficulties. As the fever subsides to normal or subnormal, the patient sweats profusely. Since the entire malarial attack or paroxysm lasts several hours, the patient is customarily exhausted and falls off to sleep. In a primary acute case the paroxysms first appear every several hours but soon stabilize at about every 48 hours. In untreated cases symptoms become less pronounced after a few weeks, but relapses may occur for years later, particularly during stress periods.

Ovale infection in a patient is similar to vivax infection except that the symptoms in ovale are less severe, relapses seem less frequent, and it responds better to chemotherapy.

The paroxysm of quartan malaria is similar to that of vivax and ovale malaria except that the onset is more gradual, and it quickly stabilizes at about every 72 hours. Relapses occur and quartan malaria may last up to 20 years in a patient without treatment. Kidney dysfunction usually accompanies this type of malaria when it is of long duration.

Falciparum is the most insidious type of malaria. The onset is very sudden, and paroxysms may run 12 to 36 hours so that one overlaps the other. If fever is intermittent, it may resemble that of vivax (peaking every 48 hours) or peak daily or even with a double rise every 24 hours. Vomiting and delirium are not uncommon. Subsequent attacks may be more severe than the first, but the infection usually runs its course after several weeks. Relapses are thought not to occur without reinfection. A very serious side to falciparum infection is fast-developing anemia, stroke, coma, heart failure and pneumonia—due to clogging of capillaries. This infection is also associated with a condition called blackwater fever in which there is hemolysis of erythrocytes and excretion of hemoglobin in the urine.

Other aspects of malaria infection, especially of long duration, include anemia and enlargement of the spleen and liver—particularly the spleen.

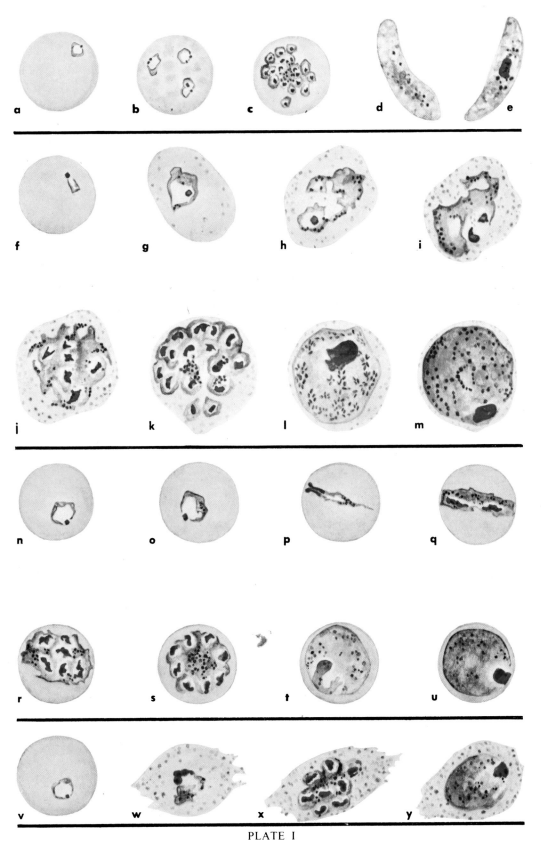

PLATE I

(*See over for legend*)

PLATE I

Human species of Malaria (From Nauck, E. G.: *Lehrbuch der Tropenkrankheiten*, 3rd Edition; Georg Thieme Verlag, Stuttgart, 1967.)

Plasmodium falciparum (a–e): a–b, ring stages; c, schizont (rarely seen in peripheral blood smear); d, microgametocyte; e, macrogametocyte.

Plasmodium vivax (f–m): f–g, ring stages; h, ameboid trophozoite; i–k, developing stages of schizont, showing mature merozoites in k; l, microgametocyte; m, macrogametocyte.

Plasmodium malariae (n–u): n–o, ring stages; p–q, band stages; r–s, developing and mature schizonts; t, microgametocyte; u, macrogametocyte.

Plasmodium ovale (v–y): v, ring stage; w, ameboid trophozoite; x, mature schizont with merozoites; y, macrogametocyte.

These organs enlarge due to increase in lymphoid tissue. Terminal malarial cases exhibit a grayish, blackish pigmentation to many organs, especially the liver, spleen, and bone marrow.

Life Cycle. Malaria is transmitted by the bite of certain female anopheline mosquitoes. The infective organisms are located in the salivary glands of the insect and are introduced into the vascular stream of a patient with the insect's bite. The malaria parasites remain in the blood for less than an hour and then enter parenchyma cells of the liver. In the liver cells the parasites undergo asexual multiplications, the progeny of which are called *merozoites*. After one to many generations in the liver the liberated merozoites invade erythrocytes and circulate in the vascular stream. This tissue phase of malaria is referred to as *exoerythrocytic* (EE), and although it does not result in symptoms to the patient, it may persist for a long time. It provides a breeding ground for future generations of parasites and is responsible for the relapse phenomenon. The lack of persisting EE stages in falciparum malaria is believed to account for the rarity of relapses.

After the merozoites from the EE stages infect erythrocytes, there occurs a multiplicative process in these infected cells. Growth, development, and eventual division takes place within each infected erythrocyte, and the red blood cell ruptures, releasing new merozoites. These parasites may then enter other erythrocytes and repeat the divisional cycle, resulting in periodic progeny and infection of red blood cells. It is when the density of infected erythrocytes reaches a certain level that the patient begins to experience signs and symptoms.

After some generations some merozoites do not repeat the multiplication process in erythrocytes, but rather develop into male and female gametocytes of the malaria organism. These sex cells are the only stages of the parasite which develop further in the mosquito when she takes blood from an infected person.

Inside the midgut of the mosquito the male and female cells mature, and there is fertilization. The progeny of fertilization eventually locate beneath the limiting membrane of the gut and develop into pustule-like structures (oocysts). By means of a series of asexual divisions many new malaria organisms (sporozoites) develop within these structures. The oocysts eventually rupture, and the released sporozoites work themselves into the salivary glands of the insect, and are introduced into a patient with subsequent bites.

The geographic distribution of human malaria is cosmopolitan. Vivax malaria has the widest range and is the species which extends into temperate zones. Falciparum malaria is found mostly in tropical and subtropical areas, and, together with vivax malaria, they constitute about 93 % of all human cases. Quartan malaria is widespread but exists in pockets in subtropical and temperate zones. The distribution of ovale malaria is spotty, and its incidence in people is usually low except in certain areas of Africa, where it is the predominant species.

Human malaria and simian malaria can be transferred one to the other under natural conditions, but to what degree this is going on in nature has as yet not been determined.

Diagnosis. Since the classical remittant chills, fever, sweats, anemia, and splenic enlargement of malaria mimic a variety of other human infections, the only completely reliable means of diagnosis is the microscopic identification of the malarial organisms from stained blood films from the patient.

Thick and thin films are preferably made on the same slide and air-dried; the thick film is dehemoglobinized with water, and then both thick and thin films are fixed in methyl alcohol and stained with such stains as Giemsa's or Wright's stain. The thick film concentrates the blood over 20 times and is used mostly to determine whether or not malaria is present. The thin film shows greater morphological detail of the parasites and is therefore used for species determination.

Since there are various morphological changes in the malarial organisms during their erythrocytic cycle, some necessary terms are applied to these changes. The study of malarial stages often causes confusion to the beginner, because it is not sufficiently emphasized that these stages do not "jump" from one to the other, but rather develop in time (as do the stages in mitotic divisions of cells). It is the intergrade developmental stages which are often difficult to interpret. In order to diagnose malaria, particularly on a differential basis, the *erythrocytic stages* must be first learned (Plate I).

Trophozoite. This term is applied to all intra-erythrocytic stages of the parasite until the nucleus divides. In the young trophozoites the parasite consists of a red, chromatic dot of nucleus and pale, bluish cytoplasm surrounding a vacuole. It is often referred to as the "ring" stage. There are many artifacts which may resemble the parasite at this stage, the most common of which are platelets resting on an erythrocyte. The young trophozoite grows, changes its shape, and evenually occupies most of the infected cell.

Schizont. This term is applied to the stage in which one or more nuclear divisions have taken place following growth of the trophozoite. There occurs multiple nuclear divisions, followed by cytoplasmic divisions. The end result of these processes is a group of new progeny (*merozoites*) making up the schizont. In early development (before the merozoites are completely formed) the schizont is sometimes referred to as a *presegmenter,* and when maturation is complete and prior to the disruption of the merozoites from the cell, the schizont is also called a *segmenter.*

Gametocytes. Although the male and female gametocytes can be morphologically distinguished, they both have an undivided nucleus and a considerable cytoplasmic mass. During the development of malaria in erythrocytes there occur granules of greenish-blackish pigment. Mature gametocytes are often confused with growing trophozoites, but the presence of more pigment in gametocytes serves as one means of making the distinction.

Falciparum malaria is indicated by a peripheral blood smear which reveals only ring stages and/or the characteristic, sausage-shaped gametocytes. The other stages most usually develop in deeper blood. Although the young trophozoite cannot always be differentiated from the similar stage in other species, the falciparum ring often has double nuclei per parasite, multiple parasites per erythrocyte, and so-called appliqué organisms hugging the periphery of the red blood cell. If the characteristic sausage of crescent-shaped gametocyte is seen (in which the outlines of the erythrocyte are barely visible or absent), then there is absolute assurance of falciparum malaria.

Vivax malaria is characterized by several features. All erythrocytic stages may be seen from peripheral blood smears, but certain ones predominate—depending on when the smear was made. Of considerable diagnostic value is the fact that with the growth and development of the vivax trophozoite, the infected cell enlarges considerably. Moreover, there develops erythrocytic stippling referred to as Schüffner's dots. An additional diagnostic feature is that the merozoite progeny of the mature schizont number between 12 to 24 and do not usually form a geometric pattern around a central mass of malarial pigment.

Quartan malaria is characterized by the infected cell's *not* being enlarged, and Schüffner's dots are absent. There are considerably fewer merozoites (7 to 9) in the mature schizont, and they are often arranged peripherally around a central mass of pigment—forming the so-called "rosette" stage. An additional criterion that is often used is that the growing trophozoite often appears as a band across the erythrocyte, in contrast to the finger-like appearance of vivax infections.

Ovale malaria closely resembles quartan in appearance, but its effect on the host cell is more similar to vivax malaria. It can be recognized by oval enlargement and fimbriation of the infected erythrocyte and the early appearance and coarser nature of Schüffner's dots. The number and arrangement of merozoites per mature schizont is similar to quartan malaria.

Although an experienced worker can quickly determine from a stained blood film what species is involved, it is good practice to observe several organisms before a definite diagnosis is made and to determine the possibility of infection with two species. A single negative blood film has no significance, and malaria cannot be ruled out until a series of blood films have been studied at 8–12 hour intervals over a few days.

Treatment. Chemotherapy and supportive measures are the course of action. There are several good drugs for malaria. The choice depends on what it is desired to accomplish.

For a clinical attack the drug of choice is chloroquine. Unless the malaria strain is resistant, this will relieve symptoms of vivax, ovale, and quartan malaria and cure falciparum infections. If resistance is encountered, a quinine regimen is indicated.

To accomplish a radical cure of vivax, ovale, and quartan infections, a combination of chloroquine and primaquine is the standard course of treatment. The latter drug has a narrow margin of safety and is often associated with acute hemolytic anemia, especially in dark races.

There are many suppressive drugs that are used in malarial zones in order to prevent clinical symptoms but *not* infection. These include chloroquine, camoquine, quinacrine, and pyrimethamine. It should be emphasized that a person on suppressive drug in a malarious zone should continue suppressive treatment (or go on primaquine treatment) when he returns to a nonendemic area (if he has infection but no symptoms). Otherwise, he will experience clinical malaria soon after he goes off suppressive treatment.

Post-Treatment Advice. The importance of suppressive drugs, the use of insect repellents, and the relapse phenomenon should be explained to the patient. Moreover, the prohibition of a malarial patient as a blood donor should be pointed out.

SELECTED REFERENCES

Alvarado, C. A., and Bruce-Chwatt, L. J. 1962. Malaria. *Scientific American, 206:* 86.

Boyd, M. F. (Ed.) 1949. *Malariology.* 2 vol., W. B. Saunders Company, Philadelphia.

Bruce-Chwatt, L. J. 1964. Changing tides of chemotherapy of malaria. *Brit. Med. J., 5383:* 381.

Russell, P. F. 1955. *Man's Mastery of Malaria.* 308 pp., Oxford University Press, London.

——, West, L. L., Manwell. R. D., and McDonald, G. 1963. *Practical Malariology,* 2nd ed. 750 pp., Oxford University Press, London.

Warshaw, L. J. 1949. Malaria, *The Biography of a Killer.* 349 pp., Rinehart & Company, New York.

Wilcox, A. 1960. Manual for the microscopic diagnosis of malaria in man. *Public Hlth. Serv. Pub. No. 796.*

World Health Organization. 1961. Chemotherapy of malaria. *Tech. Rep. Ser. No. 226.*

FILARIASIS

Bancroftian filariasis   *Wuchereria bancrofti*

Malayan filariasis   *Brugia malayi*

The filarian worms are slender nematodes which live in the lymphatic system and various tissues and cavities of the body, and blood-sucking insects transmit the infections. All species of these worms produce motile embryos (*microfilariae*) which usually circulate in the blood of a patient. Onchocerciasis is a filarial infection already considered as an integumentary parasite, and relatively minor worms will be discussed in the sundry section to follow. The account below deals with Bancroftian filariasis and Malayan filariasis, the two most important species of human filariasis.

Clinical Picture. The effects of filarid infection on a patient depend on such factors as age, number of exposures and length of residence in an endemic area, and sensitivity of the patient to the parasites.

Young children, and many patients having a single exposure, show little if any symptoms at all. Clinical cases may be considered as either acute or chronic. The general pathology is a combination of allergic reactions to worm and microfilariae metabolites and inflammatory and blockage effects of the worms due to their location in the lymphatic system.

Acute attacks of filariasis involve lymphangitis and lymphadenitis. These occur mostly in the limbs, breast and scrotal areas of the body. The affected area becomes tender, erythemic and often endematous, and the patient experiences chills and fever. The glandular enlargement may subside, and the patient later exhibits similar signs and symptoms but usually of less severe nature. A primary case showing little or no hypersensitivity is self-limiting and runs its course in a year or so.

In allergic patients the above clinical picture is accompanied by urticaria. Inflammation of lymphatics is severe to the point of blockage of the vessels. Lymph collects behind these blockages and may burst into various areas of the body. Tissues become swollen and rubbery. In extremely sensitive cases and in sensitive cases of long duration in endemic areas, certain parts of the body increase tremendously in size. This clinical state is called elephantiasis and generally takes years to develop.

The effects to the patient of Malayan filariasis are similar to those of Bancroftian filariasis except that the former is less severe.

Life Cycle. Various types of mosquitoes transmit the infection. The infective filarid larvae are released from the proboscis of the insect when it bites, and these larvae enter the vascular system. From this point until the larvae mature into adult worms in the patient, surprisingly little is known, except that it takes several months or more for full maturation of the worms and appearance of microfilariae in the blood.

The adult worms are usually tangled in lymph glands and ducts, and the females give birth to motile embryos—the microfilariae. These circulate in the blood of a patient, and if sucked up by a suitable mosquito, develop to the infective stage after a few weeks and migrate to the proboscis area.

Although microfilariae may be present to some degree at all times, most strains of filariae exhibit periodicity in that the highest density of these parasites in the peripheral blood occurs between 10 p.m. to 4 a.m. Some strains do not have periodicity.

Bancroftian filariasis has wide distribution in tropical and subtropical areas—Africa, Southern Europe, Middle East, Far East and Latin America; Malayan filariasis is confined to the Far East. In some areas the geographic distribution overlaps. Although man is the only known host for the Bancroftian type, the Malayan kind of infection is also naturally present in such animals as monkeys, cats, and dogs.

Diagnosis. Definite diagnosis is based on the microscopic identification and microfilariae from peripheral blood. The blood sample is taken between 10 p.m. and 4 a.m., and a wet preparation will reveal the active microfilariae. For specific diagnosis, thick and thin smears are stained with Giemsa's or Wright's stain and examined microscopically. The larvae are cylindrical and taper at the posterior end. Also, at the hind end can be observed a sheath which is a remnant of the eggshell. There are many nuclei in the bodies of microfilariae, but *Wuchereria* can be distinguished from *Brugia* by the fact that nuclei of the former do not extend into the tip of the tail (Figs. 58A & 58B).

In chronic cases where microfilariae cannot be recovered, skin testing and the complement fixation test are of value in determining filariasis.

Treatment. Diethylcarbamazine is active against the microfilariae but less so against the mature worms (unless given for long periods of time). Suramin is active against the adult worms and may be used before, or in combination with, diethylcarbamazine. Because the killing of microfilariae and possibly the worms may result in severe reactions

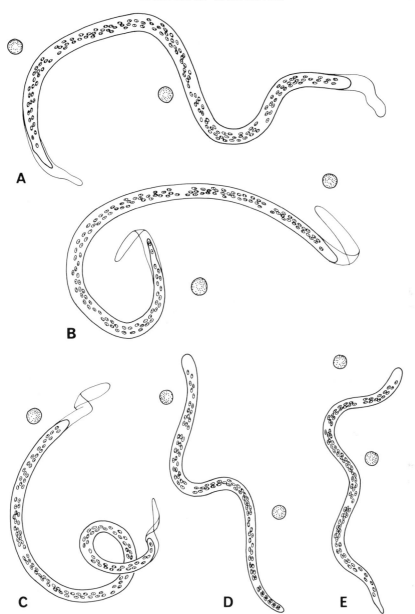

FIG. 58. Microfilariae from blood smears: (A) *Wuchereria bancrofti;* (B) *Brugia malayi;* (C) *Loa loa;* (D) *Acanthocheilonema perstans;* (E) *Mansonella ozzardi.*

to a patient, premedication with antihistamines or corticosteroids is usually advised.

Pressure bandaging and corticosteroids are used for extreme cases, and patients with elephantiasis can be temporarily helped only by surgery.

Post-Treatment Advice. A patient out of the endemic area should be reassured that the probability of his developing elephantiasis is practically nil. Persons traveling to endemic areas ought to be reminded of measures directed against mosquito bites.

SELECTED REFERENCES

Hawking, F. 1962. A review of progress in the chemotherapy and control of filariasis since 1955. *Bull. Wld. Hlth. Org., 27:* 551.

Kagan, I. G. 1963. A review of immunological methods for the diagnosis of filariasis. *J. Parasitol., 49:* 773.

Kessel, J. F. 1961. The ecology of filariasis. IN *Studies in Disease Ecology.* J. M. May, Ed. pp. 45–71. Hafner Publishing Company, Inc., New York.

Markell, E. K. 1964. Filarian infections in a California clinic. *Ann. Int. Med., 61:* 1065.

Wilson, T. 1961. Filariasis in Malaya—a general review. *Trans. Roy. Soc. Trop. Med. & Hyg., 55:* 107.

OTHER FILARIDS

Loa loa

Acanthocheilonema perstans

Mansonella ozzardi

There are a few other species of filarian worms that infect the human patient, but they are clinically less important than Bancroftian and Malayan filariasis and onchocerciasis.

Loiasis is caused by the nematode *Loa loa.* Although the adult worms move about in the subcutaneous tissues, the microfilariae of the worm circulate in the blood. The worms are noticed when they appear in the conjunctiva or move across the bridge of the nose. An infected patient exhibits edema of the eyelids and conjunctiva, as well as itchy swellings on various parts of the body. These inflammatory swellings are thought to be allergic reactions, and they eventually subside. A patient becomes infected by the bite of deer flies in Central and Western Africa. Monkeys are thought to serve as reservoir hosts. It takes several months for adult worms to develop in a patient. Diagnosis is made by the microscopic identification of the sheathed microfilariae (Fig. 58C) in stained blood films (nuclei extend into the tip of the tail). Thick blood smears are made during the daylight hours. An intradermal skin test and a complement fixation test are also useful in diagnosis but are not species specific. Treatment involves surgical removal of the worms, if possible, and/or the administration of diethylcarbamizine or suramin.

The filarid *Dipetalonema perstans,* or *Acanthocheilonema perstans,* is found in patients in parts of Africa and South America. The adults live in deeper connective tissue and the microfilariae in the blood, but except for minor allergic problems, this nematode is not considered highly pathogenic. The microfilariae (Fig. 58D) can be distinguished from peripheral blood smears. They are unsheathed, and nuclei extend into the tip of the tail.

Mansonella ozzardi occurs in various countries of Latin America. The adults live in connective and fatty tissue but apparently cause very little damage to the patient. The microfilaria (Fig. 58E) can be distinguished from other filarid worms by the fact that it is unsheathed and lacks nuclei in the tip of the tail.

SELECTED REFERENCES

Cahill, K. M. 1963. Other filarian infections of man. *New York J. Med., 63:* 1551.

Nelson, G. S. 1965. Filarian infections as zoonoses. *J. Helminthol., 39:* 229.

chapter seven

DIAGNOSIS AND TREATMENT

The very practical side of medical parasitology is diagnosis and treatment of the case. The question of deciding what parasitic infection a patient may have and the course of action one should take closely relates to satisfactory knowledge of many things—the foremost of which is the life cycle of the parasite in the body. If there is any unifying theme to the practical aspects of diagnosis, it certainly involves the life cycle. The real onus on a physician is to get a reliable diagnosis in the shortest possible time. This is related in no lesser degree to a satisfactory knowledge of the field of parasitology than the general practice of medicine is to the form and function of the human body.

A history of the patient is probably more important in the preliminaries of diagnosing parasitic infections than in other types-—especially if one is acquainted with the geographic distribution of the parasites. Such items as occupation, avocation, habits, travel (particularly to known endemic areas) offer opportunities to acquire parasitic infection, and at the same time such information may exclude being suspicious of parasites.

A cutaneous lesion on a person returning from the Middle East may certainly suggest leishmaniasis; known dirt-eating habits in a sick child may suggest nematode infections such as ascariasis and visceral larva migrans; group illness after a pork barbecue may indicate trichinosis; cutaneous lesions on a plumber who must crawl under houses should lift the eyebrows for creeping eruption.

On the other hand one would not suspect visceral leishmaniasis, African sleeping sickness of schistosomiasis in a patient who has not been out of the continental United States. The point is that one ought to have sufficient information about the general field of parasitology to permit suspicion of parasites at an early date, rather than work the patient half to death and then consider parasites as a last resort after nothing else has worked out (diagnostically speaking).

In only a few parasitic diseases are signs and symptoms suggestive of specific infection, and even these require diagnostic confirmation by some other means—so diagnosis is more of a laboratory problem than a clinical one. In this regard one ought to know that there are practically no formal courses in parasitology for medical technicians in the United States. Moreover, those responsible for technician training are usually pathologists and microbiologists who themselves are not generally prepared along these lines. This is not criticism toward any group but simply a fact which ought to be recognized by the physician requesting study of a diagnostic sample.

The question for the physician becomes at least threefold: (1) having a basis for suspecting parasites in the first place; (2) knowing diagnostic parasitology to the point of at least handling diagnostic samples intelligently; and (3) interpreting laboratory results.

It has been said that diagnostic parasitology is largely a matter of blood, sweat and feces. Whereas the microscopic examination of feces and blood is more or less routine for patients who have lived or traveled in the tropics, such has not been the practice of medicine in temperate zones. It is accurate to say that most parasitic infections can be detected by the direct examination of fecal and blood samples (the sweat is generated in working over these materials).

Stools of patients who have had barium, bismuth or mineral oil are of no value for laboratory examination of parasites, but stools normally passed, or from saline purge or enema, are acceptable.

If one suspects an acute case of intestinal amebiasis, the stool sample should be brought to the laboratory as soon as possible and arrangements made for somebody to receive it and examine it for trophozoites. If this is not possible, the next best thing is to keep the stool at room temperature or refrigerate it. The stool should never be kept at incubation temperatures, as the trophozoites do not last that way. There is no point in sending in a stool sample from a patient who has been on antibiotic therapy for some days and ask for demonstration of amebic trophozoites. At the same time nothing very admirable can be said for the physician who sends in a formed stool to be checked for amebic trophozoites; they simply will not be in the sample. A single negative stool has no significance in ruling out amebiasis, and final negative diagnosis can be made only upon several examinations over several days. The interior of a fecal mass is less profitable than the outside edge or flecks of mucous or blood.

To the *trained* person the emulsification of a little feces in a couple of drops of saline may reveal cases of amebiasis, giardiasis; nematode infections—such as ascariasis, whipworm, hookworm, and strongyloidiasis; fluke infections of *Fasciolopsis, Heterophyes, Clonorchis,* schistosomes; and most of the human tapeworm infections—which means the great majority of human parasites.

The implication is not, however, that laboratory diagnosis is simply a matter of slapping a piece of feces on a slide and peeking down the tube of a microscope. Diagnosis depends on adequate knowledge and experience with various anatomical features of the parasites. Moreover, for the laboratory worker there are numerous concentration techniques and procedures which permit both detection of light infections and the quantitation of infections. Fixing and staining procedures are also used for situations which may require critical morphologic diagnosis, as for amebae.

Other procedures for detecting intestinal parasites are often useful. Proctoscopic aspirates or biopsy taken from pinpoint lesions of the colon often reveal trophozoites of *E. histolytica.* Rectal snips are more rewarding than fecal examinations in chronic cases of schistosomiasis. The scotch tape anal swab is the diagnostic method of choice in pinworm infection and also highly rewarding in beef tapeworm infection. Duodenal aspiration is sometimes used for diagnosing some infections. There are those who feel this is the method of choice for strongyloidiasis and giardiasis cases, although the patient will rarely agree that this is true.

Blood is another valuable diagnostic sample which may be used both directly and indirectly. Its direct use is by stained thick and thin smears, and the microscopic examination of smears will reveal such infections as malaria, African trypanosomiasis, and filariasis. The indirect use of the blood sample, either by laboratory animal inoculation or serologic tests, may indicate Chagas' disease, toxoplasmosis, and trichinosis.

Biopsy (already mentioned for amebiasis and schistosomiasis) is often the only diagnostic method for determining definite diagnosis of trichinosis, hydatid, cysticerosis, sparganosis, and onchocercosis cases.

The radiograph is the least useful method in diagnosing parasitic infections, although it may arouse suspicion of hydatid disease, paragonimiasis, and cysticercosis.

Immunological procedures of diagnosis include both serologic and skin tests. While often useful in diagnosis, these tests are not usually of a high order of specificity and, with a few exceptions such as trichinosis, are not commercially available.

Excepting immunologic tests, most diagnostic methods have little value, *unless* the laboratory diagnostician has a sound morphologic knowledge of the parasite, since it must be distinguished from many other things which are forever present. Moreover, the physician must have adequate knowledge as to where in the body—and when—a diagnostic sample is best taken before being sent to the laboratory for identification.

Once diagnosis has been accomplished and clinical judgment rendered with regard to intensity of parasitic infection, degree of pathology, and general health status of the patient, chemotherapeutic decisions are in order.

It cannot be overemphasized that every time a patient undergoes chemotherapy, he is submitting to a differential toxic material. Although drugs licensed for human use have usually passed extensive tests with regard to several factors, there is probably no drug on the market which does not produce at least some transient side reactions in addition to its action against the parasite. It is thus extremely important not only to have knowledge of antiparasitic drugs, but also to be familiar with such factors as relative or expected toxicity, contraindications, and precautions in the administration of the compounds (the manufacturer's package insert gives details of these factors). Moreover, dosages and time schedules are not to be regarded lightly, since the claim for efficacy and safety are based on certain tested regimens.

The following (alphabetically listed) drugs have proved useful in the management of protozoan and helminthic infections and constitute the chemotherapeutic agents listed in the text. There are omissions, and opinions vary as to "drug of choice"—based on relative activity, toxicity, ease of administration, relative cost, availability of the drug, and whether treatment involves a hospitalized case or not. Unless indicated otherwise, the dose schedules are for adults. When children's dosages are not mentioned, they usually constitute one-half the adult figure.

BEPHENIUM HYDROXYNAPHTHOATE (Alcopar)
(5 g tablets)

Use:	Hookworm (ancylostomiasis), especially if patient also has ascariasis.
General Toxicity:	Well tolerated.
Dose Regimen:	Single 5 g oral dose on empty stomach.

BITHIONOL (Bitin)
(2 g tablets)

Use:	Paragonimiasis.
General Toxicity:	Usually well tolerated.
Dose Regimen:	2 g daily for 15 days.

CHLOROQUINE DIPHOSPHATE (Aralen)
(250 mg tablets)

Use:	Extraintestinal amebiasis; malaria (therapeutic and suppressive).
General Toxicity:	Well tolerated, but visual disturbances in some patients, especially after long-term administration.
Dose Regimen:	(amebiasis)—1 g (500 mg b.i.d.) for 2 days, followed by 500 mg per day (once daily) for 14 days.
	(malaria—therapeutic)—1 g initially, 500 mg 6 hr later, then 500 mg once daily for 2 days.
	(malaria—suppressive)—500 mg once weekly.
	When using chloroquine for extraintestinal amebiasis, also administer tetracycline and/or diodohydroxyquin for possible intestinal amebiasis.

CHLORSALICYLAMIDE (Yomesan)
(1 g tablets)

Use:	Intestinal taeniasis.
General Toxicity:	Usually well tolerated.
Dose Regimen:	1 g chewed and taken with water; repeated 1 hr later, followed by saline purge 2 hr later.

DIETHYLCARBAMAZINE (Hetrazan)
(10 to 100 mg tablets)

Use:	Filariasis.
General Toxicity:	Well tolerated, but indirectly produces allergic reactions due to allergens released from affected worms.
Dose Regimen:	6 mg per kg (2 mg per kg t.i.d.) daily, after meals for 3 to 4 weeks.

DIODOHYDROXYQUIN (Diodoquin)
(650 mg tablets)

Use:	Chronic intestinal amebiasis; dientamebiasis; balantidiasis.
General Toxicity:	Well tolerated, but not to be used in iodine-sensitive or hyperthyroidic patients.
Dose Regimen:	1.95 g (650 mg t.i.d.) after meals for 20 days.

DITHIAZANINE (Delvex)
(50, 100, and 200 mg tablets)

Use: Whipworm, strongyloidiasis.

General Toxicity: Gastrointestinal upset, especially in children; highly toxic—some fatalities in patients with inflamed gastrointestinal tract.

Dose Regimen: (whipworm)—300 mg (100 t.i.d.) after meals on first day, followed by 600 mg (200 t.i.d.) after meals for 5 days; children receive half the above doses.

(strongyloidiasis)—same doses as for whipworm, but treatment is for 2 to 3 weeks.

ETHYLSTIBAMINE (Neostibosan)
(300 mg ampules; 6 ml sterile distilled water added to make a fresh
5 % solution)

Use: Leishmaniasis, especially the visceral type.

General Toxicity: Gastrointestinal upset; not to be used in patients with pulmonary or renal disorders.

Dose Regimen: Initial 4 ml intravenous dose of 5 % solution, followed by 6 ml of fresh 5 % solution every 24 hr for 15 to 20 days.

EMETINE HYDROCHLORIDE
(ampules—150 mg in 3 ml fluid)

Use: Amebic dysentery, and liver amebiasis when chloroquine unsuccessful.

General Toxicity: General toxin, especially to vascular system.

Dose Regimen: Not more than 65 mg per day intramuscularly or subcutaneously for 2 to 3 days.

HEXYLRESORCINOL
(100 or 200 mg gelatin capsules, or in crystals)

Use: Hookworm (when *Ascaris* is also present), intestinal flukes, and high risk whipworm cases.

General Toxicity: Well tolerated, but causes superficial burns if chewed.

Dose Regimen: (orally)—100 mg per each year of age (up to 1 g —adult dose) on empty stomach following saline purge.

(high-retention enema)—saline enema followed by coating perianal region and buttocks with petroleum jelly to prevent burns; then administer 0.3 % suspension by rubber catheter (to be retained 30 min).

LUCANTHONE HYDROCHLORIDE (Miracil D)
(200 mg tablets)

Use: Urinary and mansoni schistosomiasis.

General Toxicity: Gastrointestinal upset; turns skin yellow; not to be used in kidney or liver patients.

Dose Regimen: 15 mg per kg (5 mg per kg t.i.d.) for 7 days.

MELARSEN OXIDE
(5 % solution in propylene glycol)

Use: Early and late African trypanosomiasis.

General Toxicity: Gastrointestinal upset and symptoms of arsenic toxicity.

Dose Regimen: Intravenous injection of 5 ml of 5 % solution once daily for 4 days; then after a week's interval, the same dose regimen repeated.

MEL B (Arsobal)
(5 % solution in propylene glycol)

Use: Early and late African trypanosomiasis.

General Toxicity: Symptoms of arsenic toxicity.

Dose Regimen: Intravenous injection, 3.6 mg per kg for 4 days, followed by rest of 7 days, followed by 3.6 mg per kg for 4 days.

METRONIDAZOLE (Flagyl)
(250 mg tablets)

Use: Trichomoniasis.

General Toxicity: Well tolerated, but some diarrhea.

Dose Regimen: females—750 mg (250 mg t.i.d.) for 10 days, along with daily 500 mg vaginal insert.
males—500 mg (250 mg t.i.d.) for 10 days.

OXYTETRACYCLINE (Terramycin)
(250 mg capsules)

Use:	Acute intestinal amebiasis; dientamebiasis; balantidiasis; (given alone, or in combination with diodohydroxyquin).
General Toxicity:	Possible increase in diarrhea; also, possible fungal overgrowth of gut or vagina.
Dose Regimen:	1 to 2 g per day (250 to 500 mg q.i.d.) for 5 to 10 days.

PAROMOMYCIN (Humatin)
(250 mg capsules)

Use:	Amebic colitis (given alone, or in combination with diodohydroxyquin).
General Toxicity:	Usually well tolerated.
Dose Regimen:	1.5 g (500 mg t.i.d.) for 7 days.

PENTAMIDINE (Lomidine)
(2 % solution)

Use:	Early African trypanosomiasis; chemoprophylaxis of African trypanosomiasis.
General Toxicity:	Hypotensive reactions.
Dose Regimen:	(early trypanosomiasis)—4 mg per kg intramuscularly once daily or every other day for 5 to 10 injections.
	(chemoprophylaxis)—5 mg per kg intramuscularly once every few months.

PIPERAZINE (Antepar)
(syrup containing 100 mg per ml)

Use:	Pinworm; ascariasis.
General Toxicity:	Well tolerated.
Dose Regimen:	(pinworm)—65 mg per kg (with maximum of 2 g) once daily for 7 days.
	(ascariasis)—150 mg per kg once daily for 2 days.

POTASSIUM ANTIMONY TARTRATE (Tartar emetic)
(0.5 % solution in sterile distilled water to be made *fresh*)

Use: Schistosomiasis, especially japonicum schistosomiasis.

General Toxicity: Highly toxic, affecting circulatory and respiratory systems in some patients; not to be used in patients with heart, renal, pulmonary, or hepatic disorders or in children; causes tissue necrosis if solution spills out of vein.

Dose Regimen: Slow (3 to 4 ml per min) intravenous injection of 0.5 % solution is given once daily every other day, beginning with 8 ml and increasing the volume injected by 4 ml each day until 28 ml is administered; 28 ml is then administered every other day for 9 to 12 additional injections; a syringe of epinephrine solution should always be ready in case of medical emergency due to toxicity of the drug.

PRIMAQUINE DIPHOSPHATE
(26.5 mg tablets)

Use: Radical cure for malaria.

General Toxicity: May cause acute hemolytic anemia, espeically in heavily pigmented races; not to be used following quinacrine as latter drug potentiates its toxicity.

Dose Regimen: 26.5 mg once daily for 14 days.

PYRIMETHAMINE (Daraprim)
(25 mg tablets)

Use: Active acquired toxoplasmosis; malaria suppression.

General Toxicity: Some gastrointestinal upset, but well tolerated at low doses; a folic acid antagonist.

Dose Regimen: (toxoplasmosis)—50 mg initially, followed by 25 mg once daily for 14 days; this treatment concomitant with triple sulfonamides given

3 g initially, followed by 6 g (1 g q.i.d.) for 14 days.
(malaria suppression)—25 mg once weekly.

PYRVINIUM PAMOATE (Povan)
(oral flavored suspension)

Use:	Single dose treatment for enterobiasis; lesser use against trichuriasis and strongyloidiasis.
General Toxicity:	Usually well tolerated.
Dose Regimen:	(pinworm)—5 mg per kg as single oral dose.
	(trichuriasis and strongyloidiasis)—1 mg per kg daily for 7 days.

QUINACRINE HYDROCHLORIDE (Atabrine)
(100 mg tablets)

Use:	Intestinal tapeworms; giardiasis.
General Toxicity:	Well tolerated over short term, but may cause gastrointestinal upset and mental disturbances in some patients; long term administration turns skin and eyeballs yellow.
Dose Regimen:	(tapeworms)—800 mg to 1 g (200 mg every 10 min; children receive half the above regimen; sodium bicarbonate and a little water should be given along with tablets in order to reduce the possibility of vomiting the drug.
	(giardiasis)—300 mg (100 mg t.i.d.) after meals for 5 days.

QUININE SULFATE
(300 mg tablets)

Use:	Malaria (for cases resistant to chlorquine treatment).
General Toxicity:	Various side reactions such as dizziness, cardiac irregularity and visual disturbances.
Dose Regimen:	1.8 g (600 mg t.i.d.) for 5 to 7 days.

STIBOPHEN (Fuadin)
(5 ml ampules of 6.3 % solution)

Use:	Urinary and mansoni schistosomiasis.
General Toxicity:	Gastrointestinal upset; not to be used in liver, heart, and kidney patients.

Dose Regimen: Intramuscular injection of 1.5, 3.5, and 5 ml on days 1, 2, and 3, respectively, followed by 5 ml daily every other day for 18 injections. Children receive 20 to 30 % less volume of the 6.3 % solution.

STILBAMIDINE
(100 mg ampules; 10 ml sterile distilled water added to make up a *fresh* 1 % solution)

Use: Visceral leishmaniasis.

General Toxicity: Damage to trigeminal nerve; solutions become highly toxic when exposed to light.

Dose Regimen: *Slow* intravenous injections, 2.5 ml of 1 % solution initially, followed at 24-hr intervals for 10 to 15 days of increasing doses up to 13 ml per dose; average total dose of about 100 ml.

SURAMIN (Bayer 205)
(1 g ampules; 10 ml sterile distilled water added to make up a 10 % solution)

Use: Chemoprophylactic and therapeutic for early African trypanosomiasis; onchocerosis; filariasis.

General Toxicity: Kidney irritant and not to be used in patients with renal disorders; may also cause circulatory failure.

Dose Regimen: Trial intravenous dose of 3 to 5 ml of 10 % solution for possible toxicity; then, at 4-day intervals, 10 ml of 10 % solution are given at each injection until patient has received about 10 ml total dose.

TETRACHLORETHYLENE
(0.5 ml and 1 ml capsules)

Use: Hookworm (when *Ascaris* is absent); intestinal flukes.

General Toxicity: Usually well tolerated.

Dose Regimen: Up to 5 ml maximum single dose, on empty stomach.

TRYPARSAMIDE
(2 g ampules; 10 ml sterile distilled water added to make 20 % solution)

Use: Late African trypanosomiasis.

General Toxicity: May cause ocular disorders; not to be used in patients with ocular disease, or in pregnancy.

Dose Regimen: Initial intravenous dose of 5 ml of 20 % solution, followed by 5 ml a week later; then at 15 weekly intervals doses are gradually increased to 10 to 15 ml per dose for a total dose of 160 ml of the 20 % solution.

SELECTED REFERENCES

Beaver, P. C. 1952. The detection and identification of some common nematode parasites of man. *Amer. J. Clin. Pathol., 22:* 481.

Brainerd, H., Margen, S., and Chatton, M. J. 1965. *Current Diagnosis and Treatment,* Chapters 24 and 25. Lange Medical Publications, Los Altos, California.

Gould, S. E., Hinderman, D. L., and Batsakis, J. G. 1962. Diagnostic patterns: Eggs of of helminthic parasites of man. *Amer. J. Clin. Pathol., 39:* 512.

Seaton, D. R. 1965. Advances in the treatment of tropical diseases. *The Practitioner, 195:* 507.

Schnitzer, R. J., and Hawking, F. (Eds.) 1963. *Experimental Chemotherapy.* Vol. I, 1008 pp., Academic Press, New York.

—— 1966. *Experimental Chemotherapy.* Vol. IV, 670 pp., Academic Press, New York.

Shookhoff, H. B. 1962. Reflections on diagnostic parasitology. *Trans. N. Y. Acad. Sci., 24:* 447.

Spencer, F. M., and Monroe, L. S. 1961. *The Color Atlas of Intestinal Parasites.* 142 pp., Charles C Thomas, Springfield, Illinois.

Wright, F. J. 1964. Advances in helminthology. *The Practitioner, 193:* 519.

INDEX